JUSTINE'S JOURNEY

by

JUSTINE FORREST

All Rights Reserved under the Copyright, Designs and Patents Act, 1988.
The moral right of the author has been asserted.

No part of this publication may be reproduced, copied, stored in a retrieval system, or transmitted, in any form or by any means, without the prior written consent of the copyright holder, nor be otherwise circulated in any form of binding or cover other than that in which it is published and without a similar condition being imposed on the subsequent purchaser. All images are the property and copyright of the author and/or publisher and may not be reproduced in any media without written permission.

A CIP catalogue record for this title is available from the British Library.

Published in 2013 by ThornBerry Publishing UK
Copyright © Justine Forrest

First Print Edition 2013 ISBN 978-1-909734-01-2
Ebook Edition 2013 ISBN 978-1-909734-00-5

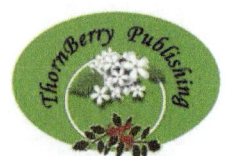

ThornBerry Publishing UK, South Gloucestershire, England
www.thornberrypublishing.com

For every single person who has suffered with obesity,

With my love

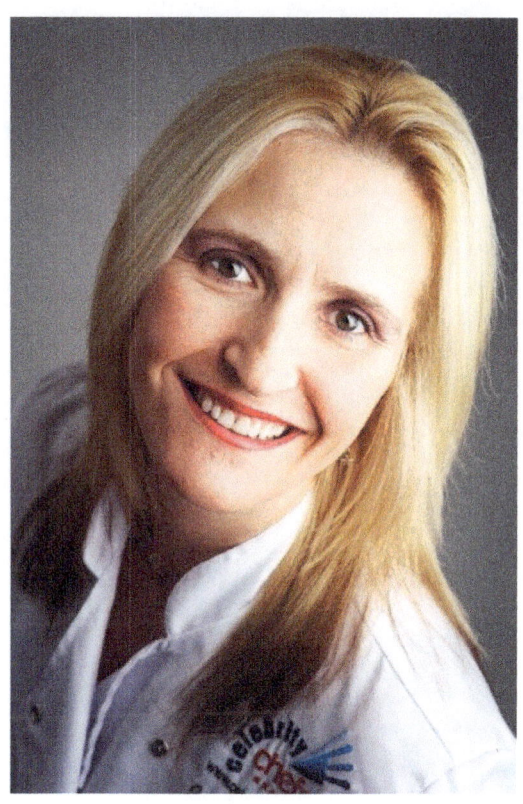

Dedication

I consider it one of the greatest achievements in my life to date to be able to dedicate *Justine's Journey* to my wonderful husband, Chris. We have certainly been through testing times but through them all Chris has always supported, looked after and loved me – fat or thin. Chris loves me for who I am and not for what I look like, and for that reason (and a million others!) I dedicate this book to him.

Disclaimer

It is always recommended that you discuss any slimming or activity programme with your doctor before you begin following this plan. Because ovens can vary, all temperatures and cooking times given are approximate and will need to be adjusted accordingly for your appliance.

Photography
www.barrymellorphotography.co.uk

Dress Design
Justine's dress on page 212 designed by
Vanity Project www.limb-clothing.com

Cover Design
David M Jones

CONTENTS

FOREWORD

AN INTRODUCTION TO MY STORY i

CHAPTER ONE 1

    How I Became a Large Lady...1

CHAPTER TWO 16

    My Family and Me... 16

CHAPTER THREE 28

    Michael Winner's Dining Stars 28

CHAPTER FOUR 47

    Surgeries and Procedures 47

CHAPTER FIVE 55

    Exercise!.. 55

        ZUMBA.. 57
        SPINNING... 59
        RUNNING 62
        SWIMMING.. 64
        ROWING 65
        KETTLE BELLS 65
        WEIGHT TRAINING 67
        CIRCUIT TRAINING.. 67
        ABS AND TONE 68

CHAPTER SIX 71

    Who is Justine Forrest Today? 71

Chapter Seven.. 78

    The Plan 78

        MY FIRST TWO WEEKS' HEALTHY LIFESTYLE PLAN 80
        GET ORGANISED... 80
        THE PLAN 81
        WEEK ONE 82
        WEEK TWO 91

CHAPTER EIGHT **101**
  Top Tips and Handy Hints 101

CHAPTER NINE **115**
  Your Very Own Journey! 115

Chapter 10 .... **123**
  Breakfasts 123

Chapter 11 .... **125**
  Light Lunches 125
    Egg Pitta 125
    Spicy Pork Burger 125
    Healthy Houmous 127
    Smoked Mackerel Pate 129
    Pitta Pizza 130

Chapter 12 .... **132**
  Healthy Teas 132
    Coronation Chicken 132
    Moussaka 133
    Spiced Sugar Roasted Salmon on a Bed of Cabbage 134
    Vegetable Kedgeree 135
    Liver, Chipolata Sausage and Bean Casserole 135
    Pork Paprika 136
    Thai Chilli Chicken on a Bed of Brown Rice 137
    Waldorf Salad 138
    Pork Ragout 139
    Spicy Chickpea Casserole 140
    Tuna Stuffed Beef Tomatoes 140
    Spiced Lamb with Couscous 141
    Shepherd's Pie 142
    Paella 143
    Honey Mustard and Chicken Pasta 145
    Penne Pasta with Chicken and Sun Dried Tomatoes 146
    Corn Chowder 147
    Chicken Rogan Josh 147
    Chicken or Beef Stir Fry 149
    Salmon and Prawn Salad and Spicy Slaw 150
    Three Bean Chilli Con Carne 151

Chapter 13 153

Healthy Snacks 153
- Healthy Fruity Flappy Jacks 154
- Healthy Honeyed Flappy Jacks 155

Chapter 14 157

Soups 157
- Spicy Butternut Squash Soup 157
- Beef and Vegetable Soup 158
- Celery Soup 159
- Pumpkin Soup 159
- Carrot and Coriander Soup 160
- Tomato and Basil Soup 161

Chapter 15 163

Super Smoothies 163
- The Energy Booster 163
- The Sexy Smoothie 163
- The Health Warrior 164
- The Brain Booster 164
- The Mood Lifter 164
- The Exercise Booster 165
- The Fat Buster Smoothie 165
- The Hangover Smoothie 165
- The Body Booster 166

Chapter 16 169

Cakes and Puddings 169
- Banana Cake 169
- Bran Cake 171
- Carrot Muffins 171
- My Basic Scone Recipe 173
- Chocolate Brownie Loaf Cake 175
- Sticky Toffee Cake 177

FOREWORD

Justine Forrest's huge weight loss literally changed her life. At 28 stones, she was unable to live normally and couldn't walk. She hadn't had a bath in years and struggled to fit into a car, and with constant hospital visits and medical worries over two of her children, Justine's weight had reached record level.

One night she had an epiphany. She realised that she would die if she didn't change her eating habits. *"I had choices, my children didn't."* She made her choice and without any help, medication or surgery, she devised a plan that would turn her life around.

In just eighteen months Justine lost a staggering 14 stones and started a career path that made her a celebrity in her home region and beyond.

Justine's Journey reveals the highs and lows, tears and triumphs and the humiliation she encountered along the way. She tells of her life-changing appearance on TV and pivotal moments that spurred her on. She reveals all the handy hints, tips, recipes and simple exercises that enabled her to shed such a massive amount of weight and keep it off.

This is a frank account of how a mum-of-three from a small northern town embarked on her epic endeavour to lose weight, get fit and start living.

Now she shares that plan with you...

Rosemary Melbourne

AN INTRODUCTION TO MY STORY

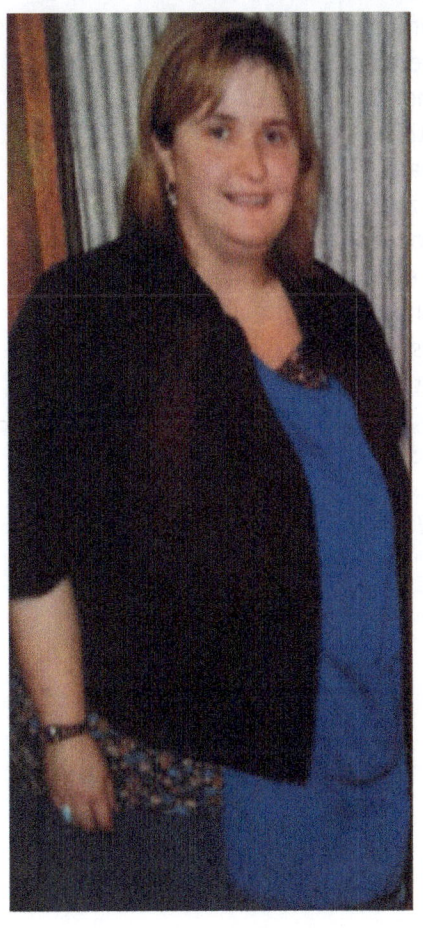

Over a period of eighteen months, I lost an enormous amount of weight. I did this all by myself with no help from any of the weight-related aids of the modern world.

At 28 stones, I was diagnosed as being morbidly obese, and I wore a UK size 32–34 in ladies clothing. Today I am 14 stones lighter and a UK size 14–16. My massive weight loss came about by a healthy eating and exercise plan. This has been an epic journey for me and my family.

If I can do it – anyone can!

Every aspect of my former life has changed and you will never know how wonderful it is living my life now, after all the restrictions I put myself and my family through for so many years. I'm no angel, nor am I special in anyway; I was just very determined that I was going to achieve it for myself this time around, having lost a large part of my life trying to diet and lose weight.

All you need is a little bit of willpower and some common sense. I truly believe that anyone can do it *if they really want to*. In my book, I tell you about myself, my family, and the journey we've been on over the last few years. I share with you the tips and handy hints that worked for me, so that you can incorporate them into your healthy lifestyle. I also share my tasty, healthy family recipes that I've created on this journey.

All this was made possible for me because of all the love and support I've had from my amazing family. Chris, my husband, never ever criticised my weight and has always truly loved me for being me. He's been the only solid thing throughout my adult life and I love him for being my soul-mate and rock. Chris has lost an incredible 35lbs too! Millie Beth, my eldest daughter, has made it possible for me to take time out of the family so I could go for long walks with our family dog, Nell, and later on in my journey to go the gym. She's watched over Alex and Christopher and made it possible for me to nip out to do some form of exercise. I thank Alex and Christopher for just being there and supporting me through some of the hard times when I've been moody, hungry and down. Everyone has really pulled together as a family, and without their support I may not have been able to do this.

I also thank Michael Winner, because without meeting him and appearing on his TV show *Michael Winner's Dining Stars*, I would never have been able to push myself and find out that I'm not useless. Through the whole experience, my confidence and self-belief have grown dramatically and I don't think now that there's any goal I can't achieve.

I've made some lovely new friends through all of my experiences and I now have a social life for the first time in years! I thank the people of Longridge too; they've motivated me at low times with their wonderful support and kind words of encouragement.

My motto: *Believe in yourself and great things will happen.*

CHAPTER ONE

How I Became a Large Lady

What it was like living day-to-day and some of the funny and humiliating experiences I had along the way.

I've never been a miserable fat person. Anyone who knows me will tell you that. Even when I've had major turmoil going on in my life, I've never carried it around with me or taken it out on other people. That's just not me.

I was the youngest of three children. My sister is six years older than me, and my brother nine years. You could say I was spoilt; in fact, my sister and brother would definitely say that! I weighed around 7lb when I was born, the average birth weight, but I started to get bigger and bigger more or less straight away. My mother said she could never fill me up; I was always a very hungry baby.

So my love of everything food began. I can remember, and also know from photographs, that from a very early age I loved peanuts. Not surprisingly, I don't like them now! But as a baby I apparently adored them and kept a glass jar for "my" salted peanuts, which I carried everywhere. I was a very generous little girl and if I thought someone had been kind or done something great, I would reward everyone and anyone with a handful of my nuts. How cute is that? But to this day, I don't understand why my parents allowed me to carry the huge glass jar around, cute or not cute. When I was three, I remember dropping the jar into my paddling pool and smashing it to bits. I then knelt on a piece of broken glass and have the proof of it today: there's a big scar on my knee. I was beside myself, but only because my nuts had gone everywhere and were all soggy and wet – it had nothing to do with the blood-stained water I was sitting in.

Being the youngest, everyone fed me and gave me sweets all the time. My mum made us stay at the dining table every night until we'd all finished all the food on our plates. She hated waste. I suppose it was because she was raised by nuns and in her early days there wasn't enough food to go around. If my sister and brother didn't like their tea, they would discreetly pass it to me under the table and I would eat everything.

My mum and dad weren't big people; they had very slim builds, especially my mum. She could, and still can, eat anything she wants without putting weight on. She's one of life's naturally slim people. Like myself, my sister and brother are taller than our parents. They've never had issues with weight gain and are both very fit and healthy. I don't think my parents ever did, or ever will, understand my issues with food. As I started to grow up, I fought against them an awful lot and at times would eat more just to spite them. Weird, I know, but as a teenager growing up, I thought that's what you did. Anything my parents told me *not* to do, I did!

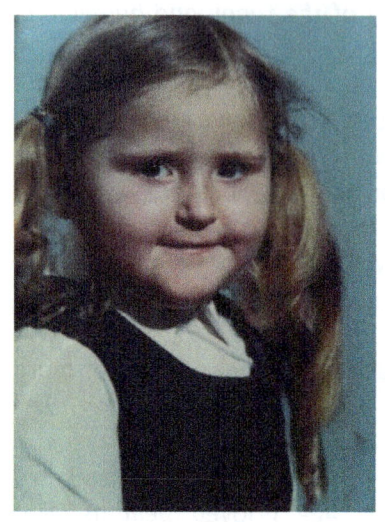

As a child, I was constantly put on "diets", and on one occasion I was taken to see the family doctor about my eating issues. My mum and dad wanted my doctor to lecture me on healthy eating and losing weight and even asked him about getting my teeth wired! This procedure, back in the mid 1980s, was the thing to do in extreme cases. It was considered a weight-loss solution for very obese people – their teeth would be wired together so they could only swallow liquids and consequently they dramatically lost weight over a short period of time. There were lots of stories circulating in the media at that time about this procedure and how amazing it was for overweight people; it was seen as the "miracle cure" for fat people. In those days, people liquidised their favourite foods so they could drink them through a straw via their wired mouth and wouldn't need to chew. It's horrifying to see the extremes people go to when they have such an addiction. Today's procedures are gastric bands or a stomach-bypass.

I was terrified of having this teeth-wiring-thingy done, but my parents really wanted me to have it and even offered to pay for it to be done privately. I had panic attacks about not being able to breath or suffocating in my sleep! What would I look like? And most important – how would I ever get my first kiss with this massive, ugly metal brace thing in my mouth, wiring all my teeth together? I refused to have it and the doctor's consultation was a complete waste of time. We came away not knowing anything about sensible weight loss or how to go about losing and maintaining a healthy lifestyle. I'm still embarrassed when I think about that time, it has stayed with me and until now, very few people knew this story about me. It really was one of the worst things my mum and dad ever suggested, and it happened at such an impressionable age too. They sent out very mixed messages. They went from one extreme to the other. On the one hand, they would buy me loads and loads of treats and junk food just to make me happy, then on the other, shout at me about what I ate and how huge I was becoming! It was so confusing. They didn't understand why I craved food and wanted to eat as much as I did.

I dread to think about the size I might have got to if I'd been growing up living in today's society, with takeaways and fast food shops on every corner. I was about nine years old when we got our first McDonalds in Southport and it was a massive treat to have a burger. Today, it's quite normal to eat take-outs every night but in those days it was a luxury, even for me.

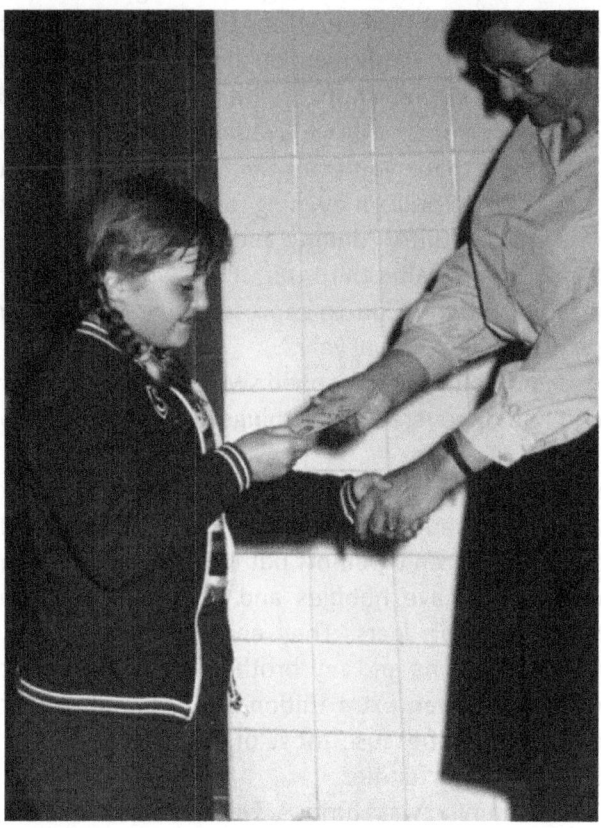

Winning my first swimming award 1978

I was sporty from a very young age and, like my brother and sister, joined Southport Swimming Club at the age of six. I followed my sister to Wigan Wasps swimming squad and swam for the city of Liverpool when I was eleven.

I loved the water and was a proper little water baby. I still enjoy swimming; it's a bit like riding a bike – once you've learnt how to do it, you never forget. Even at my largest, I always felt very comfortable once I was actually in a swimming pool, despite the nightmare of getting from the changing room to the pool – I was very self-conscious and felt everyone staring at my humongous size. My body felt so light in the water and irrespective of my size, I swam fast, with a good stroke. Swimming is such fantastic exercise and really gets the whole body moving.

Until I was fourteen, I swam every day, twice a day, the only exception being Sundays. Swimming was my life, mainly because I didn't have time to do anything else and it took over completely. I excelled in fly and backstroke, with individual medley being my strongest swim. I was thrilled to swim in the Nationals at Blackpool, for the city of Liverpool. I was only eleven then and came sixth in backstroke and seventh in fly. That was quite an achievement and I was well chuffed with myself. Our team did very well that year and we all went to a huge swimming presentation at Liverpool Town Hall. It was a big thank you from the city of Liverpool and the mayor to all our team, and was a brilliant evening for an eleven-year-old.

I also loved cross-country running and did well at school level. In my first year at high school, I came third out of the whole school in the annual cross-country race, and went on to represent my school in cross-country events throughout my high school years.

But at the age of fourteen, I stopped swimming. Teenage diversions got in the way and I had discovered other things like boys, music, being a rebel and having fun.

My mum and dad had supported me throughout my childhood with my swimming and it cost them a lot, not just financially, but with their time commitment too. We weren't well-off but Mum and Dad always thought it was very important to have hobbies and interests – opportunities they never had during the war years. They encouraged us to try all sorts of things. I had singing lessons and my brother and sister tried piano, horse riding, and water polo, even extra tuition after school. I suppose in those days we were very lucky because most of the children we grew up with didn't have the same opportunities.

Naturally, the family was furious when I decided to abandon my swimming, but life is all about choices and it was my choice to stop. I felt I was old enough to know what I wanted to do. It was a massive commitment and to this day I have no regrets about giving it up. Chris and I have been through the same thing in the last few years with our own children, but if someone isn't happy doing something, you can't make them do it.

So I stopped swimming and it isn't rocket science to work out that if you stop exercising altogether after years of intense training, and if you carry on eating the same amount of food, you'll pile on weight, which is exactly what I did.

By the time I was sixteen I was several stones heavier and to top it all off, my parents now had a fast-food takeaway shop! Unhealthy food was always at hand and as you can imagine, I made the most of it! At eighteen, I had tried every faddy diet available and some of them worked for a short while. But I wanted to lose a massive amount of weight in the shortest time possible and could never get my head around a healthy balanced eating and exercise routine.

I remember going without food for five days, living off water. *Oh my God!* What was I thinking? In general, I don't think we knew anywhere near as much about weight loss as we do today, but at that time it felt the right thing to do. Surely if you didn't eat you would lose weight? I didn't realise that when you fasted for a long period then started eating again, you literally piled it all back on and more! I did manage to lose 3½ stone during my see-saw-teens. I lived on faddy, unhealthy diets without any exercise, and at eighteen was at my slimmest and wore size 12 clothes. I felt great. I don't know how I kept this up because I skipped meals and never exercised and burnt the candle at both ends with lots of late night socialising. But of course, it eventually all piled back on, and more!

As a very large lady, life can be very difficult. At my largest, I knew that things were harder for me than your average woman and this could be something as simple as breathing.

I was always out of breath. Even on very short walks, I couldn't keep up with my family and always looked like a hot, sweaty, bright red berry. It's so strange now to think that I actually knew that my weight was seriously threatening my life. I was completely aware that my life expectancy lessened each day, and I didn't need a doctor to spell this out. I was slowly and consciously eating myself to death!

I never looked in a mirror and would avoid them at all costs. I kidded myself into thinking that if I couldn't see myself, I wasn't that big! Thinking about all the scary health risks didn't make me want to lose weight either. I was in complete denial. I never, ever went to a well-woman clinic and as soon as the letter came through the door for me to ring the surgery and make an appointment, I trashed it. I spent years thinking that it would be too hard and take too long to lose the enormous amount of weight I needed to lose, so what was the point?

I gave up before I'd even started.

We never had weighing scales in the house because they didn't go up to my weight and over the years I'd broken so many sets. I did find a set on the internet, from America (the only place you could get them from at that time), to measure my colossal weight. I knew every trick in the book to try to "lose" a few more pounds! Before heaving my bulk onto the scale I would go to the loo, then remove everything, even jewellery, to get a lower reading. I wouldn't eat for ages before weighing, or I'd move the scales to a certain floorboard to make a slight difference – anything to kid myself that I weighed less.

Over the years I was lucky not to suffer from any serious medical conditions or illnesses connected to my weight. I fooled myself that my health was good and didn't think about that side of things.

But in the dead of the night I panicked.

When the rest of the family were fast asleep, I couldn't sleep because I was so uncomfortable and couldn't find a position that eased my breathing or the pains I felt. I lay awake, scared and anxious about what I was doing to myself and my health, but even then I deceived myself and flippantly told myself: *"Well, you've got to enjoy your life, you don't drink or smoke, it's only food that you love and you could get run over by a bus tomorrow..."* And with that, I would reach for another biscuit or a whole cake I'd baked and start eating my way back to what I thought was a happy state of mind.

Something that upsets me to this day is the way people stereotype a fat person. There's so much stigma attached to being overweight and it really makes me mad. I know that overweight people have choices and could choose to eat less, but the point is that everyone is an individual and should be treated with respect. There are folk who think that fat people are second-class citizens and lower than low.

I know from experience.

For years, complete strangers would talk over and ignore me as if I wasn't there, or address me as if I'm too stupid to understand and join in the conversation. I've been blanked-out so many times, I've lost count. It's degrading and humiliating, and as a society I wish we were more understanding and tolerant. Some people perceive fat people as humans who spend their day in front of the TV, stuffing themselves with chocolate, crisps and cakes. To get to the size I was, I *did* over-eat and I'm not making any excuses, but my problem was portion control, ignorance and a complete lack of proper exercise.

I loved, and still do love, all foods – good and bad, savoury and sweet. But you can't possibly lug my amount of extra weight around and be fit. Imagine the strain I must have been putting on my heart and limbs with all that extra weight! I'm very fortunate that I didn't do myself any serious physical harm.

Fat people fall over too.

My poor children witnessed some humiliating experiences. I remember slipping in a supermarket aisle; I was flat out on the floor and was unable to heave myself up. The staff called an ambulance and by the time it arrived, Millie and Christopher were in floods of tears. The two burly ambulance men really struggled with my huge body and found it hard to manoeuvre me along. They managed to heave me into a chair and I remember saying a silent prayer of thanks that they were so strong otherwise there wasn't a hope that they could have got me upright. My ankle had swollen because of the weight and I am quite sure that, had I been the weight I am today, I would have walked out of that supermarket and no one would have been any the wiser.

On another occasion, I slipped on wet leaves and just couldn't get up. I remember the feeling of complete despair and fear as I dialled Chris's number on my mobile, while I was on the ground, but was only able to get in touch with his boss, Henry. I explained the problem and Chris eventually came to help me back up onto my feet. Weeks later, Chris told me that Henry had said to him, "Do you want me to come with you to help lift Justine?" I was mortified! People assumed that I was too heavy for my poor husband to lift – which, of course, I was!

So many embarrassing things happened because of my weight.

For many years I couldn't fit into a bath and even if I could have done, I wouldn't have been able to wash myself properly. When you're the size I was, it is a struggle to move – you can't bend to wash your feet and you have to hoist up all your rolls of fat so that you can clean under them. If you don't, you start to get sores because you sweat there so much, it all rubs and chafes and becomes very sore, so it's really important for anyone of that size to have regular washes and keep very clean. And, of course, it is impossible to reach you bum to wash there too. I didn't have a bath for sixteen years.

When I was in hospital having Millie, the doctors induced me three times, but to no avail. A nurse suggested a bath to "get things going". *That was an experience I never wanted to repeat!* I managed to fill the bath and somehow got into it, but the water got stuck behind me and created a vacuum. There was no water to the front and there was no way of evening out the water because I filled every inch of the bath. I sat there for ages and wanted to weep, I was so humiliated. It was freezing cold so I decided to get out and dry myself off, but I was wedged in and couldn't move in any direction. Eventually I gave in and pulled the emergency cord. It took two very strong nurses to somehow help ease me out. Since I've lost weight, I've become obsessed with my bath at home! Every chance I get I jump into it to lie there and relax in the warm water or do sit-ups.

My poor husband Chris had to shave my legs and cut my toenails because there was no way I could reach them. In winter, he had to put my socks on for me too, as I couldn't reach down to roll them on. God, that's love for you! Sometimes now when I'm watching the telly, I curl myself up in the foetus position – simply because I can! I can bring my legs right up and into my body, something I could never do before. I can kneel down too without my legs getting numb with pain; kneeling was out of the question at 28 stones. I used to have massive wedges of fat around my waist, shoulders and neck, and couldn't bend at all. I waddled. To touch and feel my bones now gives me great pride because I can remember a time when I just couldn't feel any bones through all the fat.

Workmen have shouted horrible abuse at me as they've driven past, and I had been turned away from a nightclub with a group of my friends. The door staff said I wasn't dressed correctly but I knew that it was because I wasn't the right image for their club. I've experienced some excruciating humiliation because of my obesity and it is only now, after losing my excess weight, that I can talk openly about it. I would never have dreamt of writing it all down or discussed it with anyone. There is absolutely nothing shocking that a large person could tell me that I haven't personally experienced to some degree. We're all in the same boat, which you soon realise the moment you start to talk to someone who is large or has lost a lot of weight. Even everyday things like going shopping.

Especially clothes shopping!

I always ordered clothes online if I could. It was so depressing to try to find clothes in the shops that fitted me. If you're a larger person, you'll know there are very limited high street shops out there for you to choose from; it may be easier now but not when I was a size 34. Most shops didn't even go up to that size, so I'd shop in the same clothes store year in, year out, where I knew they might just stock my size. I'd go straight to the back of the clothes rail and find the darkest garment in my size. It didn't matter what it looked like – as long as it fitted! Over the years it has got easier to find large sized clothes, there is more choice of style these days and online shopping helps. For years, I only wore black trousers with very long over-shirts and when I became too large for black trousers, I wore long denim skirts. I had two that fitted me, and at the end of each day I would wash my favourite one and dry it overnight ready for the next. How sad I feel now that I actually put myself through that? Today I can drag the first thing I find out of my wardrobe without worrying about the fit, and I can shop in any shop that sells clothes. It's amazing! I constantly say, "Nothing tastes quite as good as feeling and looking great in your clothes." My mum had a saying too: "A minute on your lips, the rest of your life on your hips." That's my mum for you – she's a naturally thin person who has never been heavier than 8 stone wet-through.

Another very embarrassing time in my larger life occurred when I went to visit a friend for a cup of tea and a catch-up. Visiting friends was a nightmare and something I tried to avoid; I had to ensure there was a high-backed chair to sit on. I couldn't sit on a sofa or couch – anything too low was impossible for me to get up from. In fact, I had to be helped to my feet. It was okay at home because I could roll myself slowly off the sofa and lumber to my feet. So undignified! But it worked for me.

My friend proudly showed me the lovely new chair that she'd bought for her husband on his birthday. It had two sculptured wooden legs that met underneath at the back, a bit like a modern day rocking chair. I duly admired it but kept my distance, I was happy on an upright chair that could cope with my weight. My friend said, "Try hubby's new chair, it's really comfy – he loves it!" She insisted that I sit on it. Her husband was a very large man himself and she assured me that the chair took his weight easily. As soon as I sat down, it snapped. I couldn't get up and had the bottom of the chair wedged into my bum. My friend was hysterical and all of our five children started giggling too. My face burned with shame and I was the only person not laughing, it wasn't funny! I was *so* embarrassed and it was a long time before I visited again.

One year we ordered new furniture, a two- and a three-seater sofa in lovely brown leather. When they arrived I noticed that they weren't the colour we'd ordered, so I rang the shop and they re-ordered the correct colour. But it was Christmas time, the factory was busy and they told us to keep these until the new ones arrived in a few weeks' time. In the meantime, I sat on the three-seater whereupon it made a large snapping noise in the middle and sunk to the floor. *Oh the shame!* It was replaced, but I never sat on our three-seater again, only the sturdy two-seater was strong enough and I filled that.

After our son Christopher was born I suffered badly with backache, especially through the night. I couldn't get comfortable in bed and couldn't sleep because of the pain. I lay there thinking I could die of a heart attack at any moment, because of what I had become. By morning I would be doubled with pain and Chris would massage my back for me, to enable me to get out of bed. We eventually decided to buy a new mattress, thinking that would make my back problem better. The sales assistant at the shop was full of advice and recommended a suitable mattress – which turned out to be the most expensive one in the shop! I suppose it was hope that my back problem would be instantly better; we were so gullible. Surprise, surprise... No difference! My back pain continued. The mattress was great but the problem was clearly my weight and how all that bulk pressing on my body and spine through the night made me so uncomfortable. Of course, as I started to lose the weight, my backache got better and better – it lifted like a miracle!

Another unpleasant subject to mention is how I suffered with piles. Haemorrhoids: those unpleasant vascular structures in the anal canal. I was in agony; they were always swollen and inflamed but I didn't realise that it was all to do with my diet and being obese. It only dawned on me after I'd lost all the weight that I'd completely stopped using the creams and potions and I've never suffered since.

I was covered in boils too, all over my body. Boils are raised reddish swellings, formed by bacterial infections and are very sore to touch. I had them for years, even on my bum, but they were worse on my stomach and under my bra line. They left scars which I have to this day. I thought I had gout too as there was always a red blush made up of tiny red veins around the bottom of my right leg. My doctor did tests and it wasn't – just skin problems from all the weight.

Reunions were a nightmare. I avoided them at all costs, simply because I was mortified by my size and didn't want others to see me. The thought of seeing people after a long period of absence horrified me. I hated the way I looked and dreaded the gossip when friends from the past saw my ballooning body.

Every autumn I would start another fad diet, in the hope that after a couple of months of cutting down, I'd look marginally better by Christmas. But when the party season came round (not that I did much partying because I was so self-conscious and hardly went out), I would pile the weight back (and more) in half the time it took to lose. A complete waste of time but an annual ritual, year in, year out! I thought it was a "quick-fix diet for Christmas" and I'd feel better about myself, but I ended up feeling worse. Shopping for Christmas treats began in September and I'd fill our kitchen cupboards full of supermarket offers. There were two large cupboards in the kitchen that I named *The Christmas Cupboards* in readiness for all the rubbish that I just had to buy because it was Christmas and we may get surprise visitors. *The Christmas Cupboards* were filled to bursting point and had to be restocked at least half a dozen times before the big day... You've guessed why – all that temptation! I couldn't keep away. By January and I was back to square one again with a few more extra pounds. I always equated special occasions and celebrations with providing nice food for everyone and spoiling them – most of all myself.

I gave a friend a lift recently and as she settled into the front seat she commented on how much room there was between the seats. Apparently she used to feel as though I was sitting on her knee, there had been so much of me spilling over! Chris said that whenever he drove and I sat in the passenger seat, my bulk completely covered the handbrake. I never accepted a lift with any of our friends; I knew that even if I managed to get into their car I wouldn't be able to fasten the seat belt. I always ended up doing the driving and had to wedge my tummy in, it was very painful as the steering wheel dug into my flesh.

On our first family holiday abroad to a friend's villa in Spain was a nightmare too. I'd heard so many stories about people being rude to larger people on flights and it made me nervous. Chris sat next to me and the children behind us. The stewardess told everyone to fasten their seatbelts. I went into complete panic – the seatbelt didn't fit! I was riddled with embarrassment because I was seated next to someone I didn't know and was only too aware that they could see me struggling. I had to ask the stewardess if she had a seatbelt extension. She went to check but didn't have one. When they came around to check that all the belts were secure, I looked away and didn't make any eye contact with the stewardess; I held the end of my belt in my hand so it looked as though it was attached at the other end. The holiday was ruined because I worried about the journey home and going through the seatbelt humiliation once again. *Never again!* I vowed. I wouldn't put myself through such humiliation and shame, but you soon forget. It's a bit like childbirth; you don't want to remember it – until the next time! I think that might have been the reason why we've never flown since. The fear of that embarrassing situation has always stayed with me.

It's really funny how easily I can forget things. Things that are locked away in my head until I happen to revisit old situations, then I remember something else about how hard my old life was when I was so big. There are just too many situations and experiences to remember here, but one thing for sure is that if you, the reader, empathise with me even only slightly, then it's time to make those changes and start living – this isn't a dress rehearsal, this is your one and only life. You need to live it and not waste a second of it, as I did. All those family holidays to Center Parcs – for years and years I couldn't hire a bike for myself because I was too big. All those wasted family times that we could have got so much more out of if I hadn't been so big. I liked swimming when we went on our holidays, but it was so embarrassing as I waddled to the pool. I thought everyone was staring at me and judging me, and of course, they were. I can tell you there wasn't much relaxation and enjoyment at those times. I should have been enjoying myself with my family but I was so unhappy about my weight. I've recently invested in a new racing bike, as I'd love to do a triathlon (another thing on my to-do list!). In my large years I never rode a bike; now we cycle together as a family. I would never in my wildest dreams have imagined doing that.

We recently visited our good friends Nik and Simon, and I nipped to their small downstairs toilet. It's a cubicle with a sliding door, and as I came out it hit me that I never used that loo in the past because the first time we visited I got stuck! It took me ages to squeeze out. I never used it again as I was scared they'd need to remove the door to get me out.

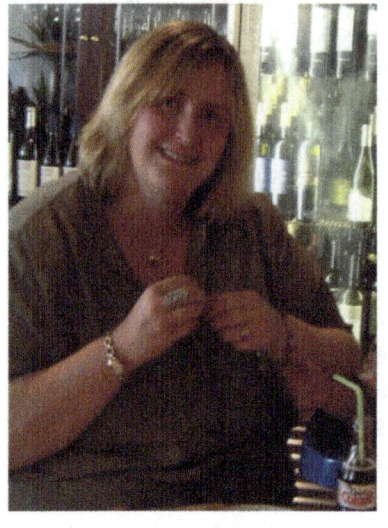

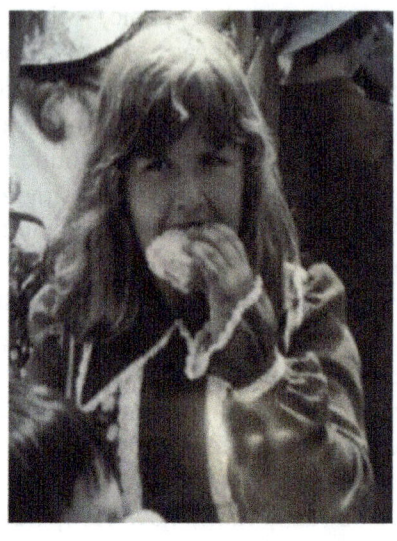

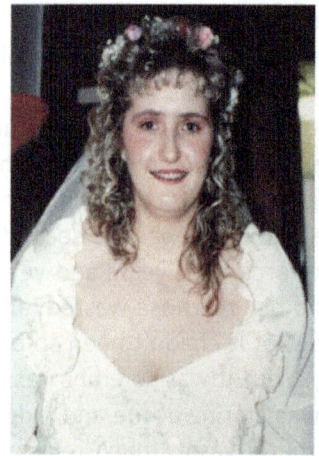

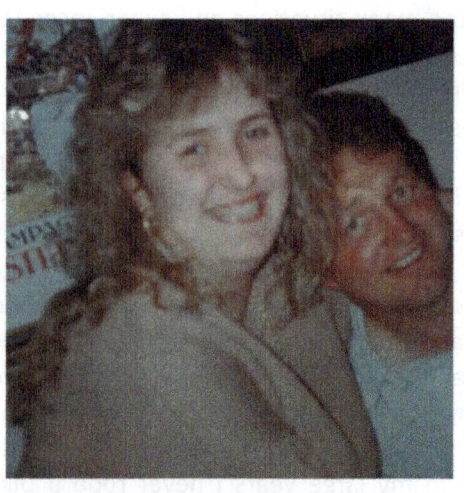

I was living my life as a prisoner in my own body

Stairs were also an enemy. Each day I would have an afternoon nap because I was so exhausted (and probably because I didn't sleep at night). If I didn't get a nap for an hour or two, I would spend the rest of the day like a zombie, I was so exhausted. In the morning, I would take anything I was likely to need downstairs – there was no way I could manage going back up the stairs until I went to bed. In the morning I would wheeze down then not go back up until bedtime because I found stairs too hard. All day I would use the downstairs toilet. Crickey, I don't know what I'd have done if we hadn't had two: maybe a bucket in the corner of the room? Ugh!

Summertime and hot weather were difficult because I lived in cardigans and big coats. I told myself nobody could see my size if I covered it. I would be very over-heated and red from wearing so many layers. I always had bruising on my tummy and legs as I underestimated gaps or space and banged into things, leaving marks on my body.

I was living my life as a prisoner in my own body, all self-inflicted I know, but still very awful for a woman of such a young age with such a young family; in fact, it's truly awful for anyone to live their life as I once did. Ask yourself that question and answer it honestly, because I don't believe that if you are overweight to the extent that I was, you are really happy. I have never, ever, met a really big person who is completely happy with the way they are.

Since losing my weight I have so much more energy and feel amazing, I have a happy body and a happy mind now for the first time in my life. I've taken control back from a situation that was spiralling out of control and I now feel truly healthy and content in myself. I have so much more confidence and I'm very happy in my own skin for a change. Nowadays, I never sleep in the day and I'm lucky if I get seven hours sleep at night because I never stop and never want to. I want to experience as much as I possibly can. Life is for the living and I want to live it all. I missed out on so much before, I now want to make up for it. I know for sure it's primarily because I've lost so much weight and also it's because of my healthy diet and exercise regime, which I'd class as a normal one and not an obsessive one. I want to eat healthy, fresh foods and take regular exercise: I work that into my lifestyle and the benefits really do show.

I remember if I was ever on my feet for a long period of time my ankles would swell up for days and I would be so tired from doing a little extra work. Over the last three years I have also not had one cold or been ill in any way, when others have been dropping like flies around me. I put that down to being able to fight the bugs off myself because I'm happy and fit and stick to a healthy diet, and sometimes that's not always about the types of foods you're eating, as much as the *amount* of food you're eating. I do think you can eat almost everything but it's more about how much of it you eat: *portion control* is the biggie. Don't get me wrong, I'm not perfect, I still have lumps and bumps in all the wrong places, but I'm happy with them because I now realise that happiness comes from within. However much I diet and workout there are always going to be those imperfections – everybody has them – that's my body shape and I'm very proud of my body shape, it's mine! I'm never going to be skinny or want to be either, it's just not my build. But that's okay because I'm happy with myself after all these years. I've learnt to love what I have and be confident with myself. I'm fit for the first time in a long, long time and I know I eat well. I'm now rising to every challenge and trying to experience all the things I missed out on over the years because I was simply too big and had no confidence in doing them. My life has completely changed and all for the better.

Since starting to write *Justine's Journey* lots of huge things have been happening in my life and I've had to be very strong to deal with these things, some good, some not so good. Some have tested my strength as an individual and as a mummy to the limits. There have been things that we've been through as a family that have been touch and go at times. All of these situations have been dealt with very differently from the way the old me would have dealt with them. I've experienced times when I've needed food as a crutch once again or because the circumstances I have been in have meant eating healthy and regularly just hasn't been that important at that time. At my worst, when I had to deal with our precious son undergoing more open heart surgery and suffering multiple life threatening complications, food and exercise didn't even enter my head. I ate what I wanted, when I could get it. I made a conscious decision not to beat myself up about it, and when eventually our son Christopher came home, I would deal with it then and get my life back on track.

Looking back now I wouldn't have done it any differently; I knew when things settled down I would go back to my lifestyle of eating well and exercising. All my friends go to the gym, that's part of my social life, I love it. But back then at those dark times I had a job to do and that was to look after my baby boy and to nurse him back to good health. I needed to have my comfort food, I may always have that addiction at tough times, but these days I know how to handle it and how to pull it back.

From where my journey is now, I often pinch myself. In the three years since losing my weight there has been lots of surgery for our family. I've had three big operations for skin removal surgery. Millie has had another operation on her cleft lip and palate and Christopher underwent his biggest open heart operation to date. All that mixed in with lots of other family appointments and procedures and bits and bats of rubbish that everyday life throws at you. Then there's all our children's activities, my writing, baking and demonstrations, and not to forget my hubby, the main man of the house and his busy schedule too. I haven't even started on the charity work and all the running with my amazing hubby.

Life really couldn't get much busier or better and none of this would have been possible in my larger lady days.

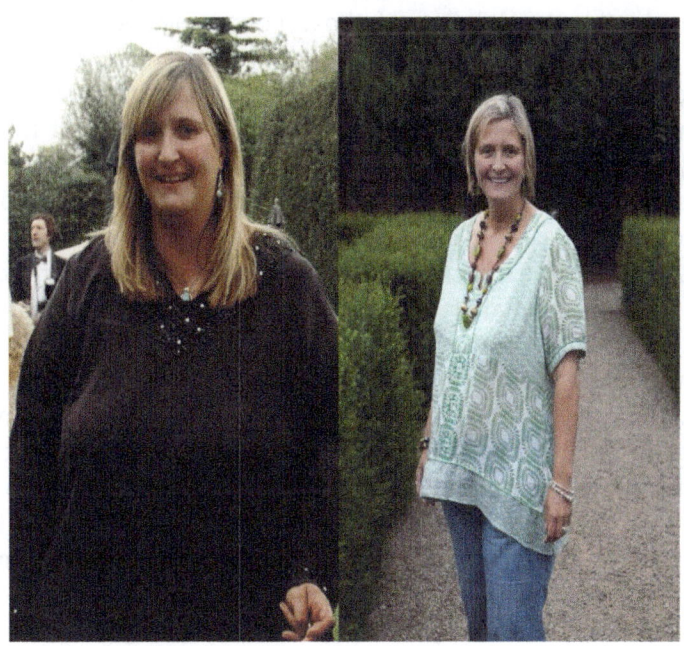

CHAPTER TWO

My Family and Me

I started working at the Ribchester Arms when I'd just turned eighteen. At that point in my life I was at my slimmest but only because I lived off fresh air and cigarettes. Skipping meals and sleep were the norm. The only exercise I got was walking up and down the bar at the Ribchester Arms, pulling pints and serving customers. I worked as a waitress too. It was one of the best jobs I've ever had, being paid to be chatted up by hot young men – who wouldn't enjoy it? One of those hot young men was my future husband, Chris, whom I met while serving him pints of beer every night. We started going out when we were both nineteen and we got engaged on my twentieth birthday. Chris has always been the one consistent thing in my life. Everyone who meets him loves him, he would do anything for anyone, and that's one of the many reasons I love him and cherish our life together. I am one lucky lady!

Chris has never, ever, criticised my size and has always loved me for who I am and not for what I looked like. I do take the mickey out of him now by saying, "It's your fault that I got so big and stayed that way for all those years. If you'd nagged me, I would have done something about it a long time ago." I'm only kidding, as there is NO WAY it would have made any difference. In fact, it might have made me eat even more, after going through those similar experiences with my mum and dad for all those years. If Chris had nagged me, I wouldn't be with him now. I couldn't live with someone that picks on you and calls you names, thinking it will encourage or shame you into losing weight – no way!

I had steadily put on weight throughout our marriage. Some would say through contentment, I would say through eating way too much. After two years I found out I was pregnant. I was very relieved as weighing 20 stone plus, I thought I'd struggle to get pregnant naturally. We were so happy when we found out. I remember the night I did my pregnancy test when the blue line came up in the positive window, we were in disbelief and rushed out to buy another two pregnancy kits from the all-night chemist in Preston. When the results were the same as the first kit, we knew it wasn't a mistake. We were going to be parents! We kept our pregnancy a secret for two weeks, as we were about to go on holiday with friends. Before we flew, I did get checked out by the doctor and booked myself in for a midwife's appointment on my return.

From the minute I found out I was pregnant everything changed. I suddenly started to control what I ate and limit fizzy pop and my cake intake to a bare minimum. I was so grateful I could get pregnant that I was willing to do anything for our baby. I made a massive effort to be as healthy as I could, as I no longer just had myself to look after; I had our baby growing inside of me and I didn't want anything to go wrong. I even started losing a little weight and doing some gentle exercise. I was feeling flipping fantastic and excited. We'd always wanted children, although Chris said if it wasn't possible then spending the rest of our lives together would be just as wonderful for him. If we could have children then Chris always wanted a dozen. *Jezzzzz!* I, on the other hand, always dreamt of having just three. We had a fabulous time with our friends in Lanzarote; all along we kept thinking it would be our last holiday before we had our family.

Upon our return, we invited all of Chris's family around for a big barbeque. All my family lived in Scotland so I had to break the news to them over the phone. My mum had been nagging me to start a family so you can imagine how excited they all were about our wonderful news. After our barbeque, I went into the kitchen and brought out our best crystal champagne flute glasses, which had been given to us as a wedding present. On the way into the garden I dropped the whole tray of glasses and smashed the lot, I was so nervous. We announced our wonderful news and Chris's dad shouted out, "Make sure it's a guddun' this time." Chris's dad had, up until then, three granddaughters, and was absolutely obsessed with us having the first Forrest grandson and carrying on the family name. Chris was always his father's golden boy, so he really wanted Chris to give him the first boy of the family.

My father-in-law was totally "Old School", and he was so proud of Chris and myself and how we coped with all the problems with our children. I've often wondered (he died a few years ago) what he would have made of all this today. We've changed so much and come so far. He would have loved being a part of all this and watching everything we've been up to, including mine and Chris's weight loss and all the telly stuff, as well as how well our little boy, Christopher, has come through his operations and everything Millie and Alex have accomplished too. He used to love to tell everyone about our children. He was a very proud granddad indeed. We used to have all the family gathering at our home, as I was the only one in the family that enjoyed entertaining and the only one who could cook too – that always helps! Chris's parents loved coming to us, they really appreciated all the trouble we used to go to even though it wasn't easy entertaining people sometimes, but without us organising everything no one else would have bothered, and we took pleasure in the way Chris's mum and dad enjoyed it all – that's what life's all about, memories and making them.

Not long after our big bbq announcement, I think it was about two weeks later, I woke in the middle of the night. I was bleeding. As I got to the bathroom I miscarried on the floor. Chris rang the hospital and they told him to bring me straight in. At the hospital they scanned me and told us I had lost our baby and offered me a D&C (Dilation, or Dilatation & Curettage – a procedure to gently scrape the lining of the uterus and remove anything that has been left behind after a miscarriage). So within hours I had gone from being very pregnant to not being pregnant at all. It had all happened so fast and we were numb.

They tell you to wait at least three months before trying for another baby and I think they were the longest three months of our lives. Everywhere I looked there were pregnant women, and it was a very hard time for us. It leaves you so empty plus the not knowing whether you'll ever be able to have any babies of your own. I remember a family member telling me that ninety per cent of all miscarriages were caused because the foetus had abnormalities. *Was that supposed to make me feel better?* The thought of our baby being disabled filled me with horror! Three whole months dragged by and I couldn't seem to stop comfort eating, I ate more and more just to try to take the pain away. Then the very first month of trying for another baby, I got pregnant straight away with Millie. Unlike my previous pregnancy, when I started to watch what I ate and exercised, I totally gave up. I thought: L*ook where that got me? If you're going to miscarry, it's going to happen whether you're being healthy or not!* I thought it had nothing to do with how fit or unfit you are.

Before Millie was born I suppose you could say I'd had a relatively sheltered life – no family deaths or any type of problems in general. So when our precious little baby girl was born with so many medical problems, I found it hard to handle it and went into a bubble for years to come. Life was very hard for me after having Millie and I also struggled with the way my life had totally changed: from working full-time and doing lots of things as a couple, I was then a full-time stay-at-home mummy with a precious baby girl who needed lots of extra care. I always considered Millie's first few months as being the biggest test in our lives and felt robbed of that new exciting first baby, mummy and child experience.

With each pregnancy, I got bigger and bigger, heavier and heavier.

Seventeen months after Millie was born, I gave birth to our second daughter, Alex. When I gave birth to Alex, aka Rapunzel (I call her that because she has the most amazing long blonde hair you'll ever see), my faith in humanity was restored. For a time Chris and I thought you were lucky to have a fit and healthy child and that the chances of that were very slim – we only thought that way because of all the time we had spent nursing Millie through her operations and hospital appointments. Seeing so many children suffering with different medical problems really made us sit up and think. Then, four years after having Millie, I gave birth to Christopher and our lives were tested once again when everything was put into perspective for us.

At my thirty-two week scan with Millie, we had discovered that she was going to be born with a cleft lip and pallet, so for the following pregnancies I was given extra scans throughout and diabetes tests because my body mass index was very high and that could mean extra complications for me and my baby. In a way, that is the only time in my life that being massively overweight has helped me. In fact, I'm pretty sure it saved our son's life, because without those extra scans they wouldn't have discovered Christopher's heart condition, which could have led to major distress and complications soon after his birth and possibly death.

We knew about Millie's condition from my thirty-two week scan and did everything we could to prepare ourselves for her birth. When they eventually gave me an emergency C-section and delivered our gorgeous baby girl, we were the happiest mummy and daddy alive. After going through ten weeks of worry, it was all over and Millie, we thought, was perfect in every other way possible. But at a day old, Millie started fitting and was rushed to the neo-natal department of the hospital where she spent the next week of her life on medication. Eventually Millie's fits stopped and we went back to the ward, then home from there. Millie never fitted again and she came off her medication a couple of months later. The first few months of her life were taken up with lots of medical appointments, and at five months old she underwent her first cleft lip operation, followed four months later with her next one. Millie has so far undergone eight corrective surgeries, with more to come in the future, if she decides she wants them.

Amidst all that, our health visitor noticed Millie had development problems down the left side of her body and sent us to a special childcare centre to be checked over and assessed. The results came back that Millie had left side hemiplegia, a form of cerebral palsy which affects the whole of her left side, from her face to her toes. Millie's CAT scan came back with news of shrinkage on the right side of her brain. I don't know how I managed to drive home safely on that awful day. Once we got over the shock of Millie's test results, we started to accept all that comes with her condition and get on with our lives. Millie was a very late crawler and walker because of her cerebral palsy but she always got there in the end. Like everything Millie does in life, it's done with strength and acceptance and she really is an inspirational girl. We're so amazingly proud of all her achievements, whether they're big or small. Everyone that meets our Millie is inspired by her approach to life.

Millie was four and Alex was three when Christopher was born and as I mentioned, we knew about his condition from the thirty-two week scan, the day after Chris's thirty-first birthday. Everything had started off so well and then the same thing happened as when I was being scanned for Millie at that same stage of pregnancy. The nurse scanned me for what seemed like a lifetime then said, "Just wait there, I'm just going to find a doctor and he can just check your scan over, just precautionary!" When she left the room I knew straight away that it was going to be something bad because it had happened the exact same way as Millie's scan. When the nurse and the doctor came back, they also had Chris with them. I was in floods of tears at this point. After scanning me again, they said there may be a problem with my baby's heart.

Chris and I were ushered into a side room to wait. When the doctor came back to see us, he had two nurses with him this time; something felt really, really bad. They explained to us as best they could what they thought was wrong with my baby's heart and said that they had made me an appointment at St Mary's Hospital in Manchester for the next day. We came away from that scan not knowing what was actually wrong, only being aware that it was very serious and life threatening.

The next day we set off at 5:30 a.m. to beat the morning traffic so we could get to Manchester in time for my appointment, which had been made for very early that morning. When we got to Manchester, I can remember we were both so emotionally drained with all this stuff going on in our heads, Chris tried to catch some sleep in the hospital car park before we went in to see our consultant. When you're faced with something horrific, you struggle to find the words to talk at times and I felt my only friend was food, as it didn't talk back or argue and it made me feel good for a short period of time.

At that appointment, the specialist explained in detail about Christopher's heart condition and his prognosis, using various scenarios. We were left alone for a few minutes for everything to sink in and for us to discuss the option of a termination. *A termination?* When I could feel my baby kicking away at me all the time! I was numb. We talked through what it would mean at that stage of my pregnancy, and looked at each other and agreed we had got through everything that Millie had wrong, so how could we give up on this baby? To this day we always say Millie actually saved her brother's life. For without experiencing everything we had with Millie, Chris and I both agree we may have taken the heart consultant's advice and terminated my pregnancy because, at that stage, Christopher's fight was only just beginning, and *if* he were to make it even through his birth, he had a very long journey to make. We came home and tried to get through

Christmas for the sake of Millie and Alex, but I knew it wasn't good news from the fact our house looked like a florist, as we received flowers from all our family and friends with their sympathy attached.

I don't know how we managed to get through the final six weeks of pregnancy with the knowledge Christopher might not make it, and even if he did survive, he could live the rest of his life going through major surgery and medical problems. They had told us that if he survived everything, his life expectancy could be anything up to 40 years.

Naturally, I turned to food for comfort once again, and would spend all day every day in bed under the covers, hiding away from the reality of everyday life. I'd drop Millie off at school every morning then go straight back to bed, leaving Alex to play in my bedroom all day with me supervising from my bed. Looking back, I know now that I was depressed and I really should have sought some help as I was sinking lower and lower into a deep depression which couldn't have been any good for my unborn baby's health, but when you get that low I suppose you're the last person to realise it.

The day of Christopher's birth eventually arrived and after another C-section our beautiful bouncing baby boy was born. We had been told there was a chance he may also have Down's Syndrome, so when he arrived into this world they rushed him off to St Mary's special baby unit, and I was left once again empty as I hadn't even seen our son in person.

The moment Christopher was born, Chris had leaned towards me and said, "I want to call him Christopher, after me, in case he doesn't make it." So, from a Jake he became a Christopher. I'm very pleased to be able to moan about the fact that it causes so much trouble having two Christophers in one house, and I always make a point of calling Christopher, Christopher. I hate it when people call him Chris, as we already have a Chris in the family and, at times, living with two Christophers does get very confusing.

Going through what we did with our precious son, Christopher really put everything else into perspective and our lives have never been the same. I would like to think, though, that if we could have had our children and sailed through everything with no worries or medical problems etc, that we as people would be the same people we are today. But I can see how these things can change you and make you the person you are, but hey ho, as they say, these things are sent to try us!

We stayed in Alder Hey Children's Hospital in Liverpool for the first nine weeks of Christopher's life, while they tried non-surgical procedures to stimulate and try to grow the right side of his heart. None of which worked. In the end, at eight weeks old, he had the first of his life saving heart operations. I found my solace in food. Days were long, lonely, very boring and completely draining. I wasn't sleeping well – I was carrying around an enormous amount of anxiety. The last thing I was thinking about was *"me"*.

When we finally brought Christopher home after those nine weeks, it felt like a lifetime since we'd been away. One of my closest and dearest friends, who had kept me going by visiting me every Wednesday night at hospital without fail, had decorated the outside of our house with lots of helium balloons to welcome us home. That is a very special memory I'll always have of our homecoming.

Over the following weeks and months I found it difficult to adjust back into a normal life. Caring for two children with special needs was very difficult, and living with a child who has a life threatening medical condition was extremely terrifying at times. I think seeing your children suffer and go through so much pain is the worst thing in the world for any parent to witness. Knowing you can't take their pain away is horrendous and I would have changed positions with them in a heartbeat. I went to my doctor at one point and was prescribed antidepressants to try to ease the burden. I only took them for a month as they didn't help in the slightest, and I was actually quite nervous about staying on them long term with all the side effects. A friend of mine had taken them and lost stones in weight. She put it all down to being on antidepressants, so that was one of the reasons I wanted to try them out, thinking they could be good for my weight loss! Of course, I didn't lose any weight, so I stopped taking them altogether. With hindsight, what I should have been doing was trying to lose weight by myself, as being so overweight wasn't helping my depression. Being my size and weight was only adding to the rut I was in. The extra weight of lugging car seats and all the other baby things around with me really took its toll on my back and joints and I was always taking some form of pain relief for the pain.

We were constantly told Christopher wouldn't thrive because of his condition but he's done amazingly. Apart from when he's been into hospital, he's never needed oxygen at home, he was even breast fed, which is rare for a baby with his condition as the breast can be an obstruction in the mouth stopping him to breathe properly. We believe we've been incredibly lucky with our children. We always take the positives out of life by thinking that Millie's damage to her brain could have meant that she would have to spend all her life in a wheelchair and she could have had learning difficulties too. Christopher, well, he might not have made it and there has always been a chance he may have suffered major health problems and lived a very restricted life indeed. So all in all, if you take all that on board, how lucky are we!

Over the next eight years, Christopher underwent another massive heart operation and many other tests on his heart and treatments. Millie has also undergone many other treatments and surgeries too for her cerebral palsy and cleft lip and palate. In one week we can have as many as seven hospital appointments! It's been tough at times when I've been away from home for long periods of time, living out of a hospital room with one of the children. All my family live in Scotland and the distance and travelling is really difficult. Chris doesn't have any family, his parents passed away a while ago. They did live near but weren't involved with our family. To be fair, we've always rolled as our little unit and have never had or asked for any help from our families. That's just the way it's always been and I think because of that it has made us stronger and closer as a family unit.

Alder Hey Children's Hospital in Liverpool is the best hospital with the kindest nurses in all the world – well, that's our opinion. Christopher was born with a congenital heart defect and has been in and out of Alder Hey Hospital for treatment and operations all his short life. He usually has his six monthly check-up at our local hospital with a consultant who has seen him since birth. I put most of my weight gain down to comfort eating, which I've done all my life in stressful situations, and on this hospital visit I made a pact with Christopher that I was going to join him and go nil by mouth. I wasn't hungry in the slightest; maybe it was because it had been another roller coaster trip to the hospital, like they always seem to be. We arrived just before 7:00 a.m. to be admitted onto K2 ward, and found ourselves experiencing a mini miracle!

    Christopher had been deteriorating in health over the last few months – nothing major, just more blue and breathless than usual. We had taken him back to see his consultant at Preston and they'd sent us for more checks at Alder Hey. They wanted a clearer look at Christopher's heart so they could map out his next operation. He was in the middle of a three-stage procedure and they thought he may need the next stage soon. Anyway, we kissed him goodbye at the hospital theatre doors only to be hunted down ten minutes later by a nurse from his ward. We had the shock of our lives, thinking something awful had happened in theatre as we were rushed back onto the ward.

    One of Christopher's surgeons met us there with another consent form. He went on to explain how they wanted to put a camera down his throat instead of what they were going to do, because they thought if they blocked the hole up that was in one of his arteries then he might not need further surgery, and they think there is a 70/30 per cent chance of success. To me, in black and white terms that means so much more, that in itself is a mini miracle! If Christopher has his third stage Fontan procedure and that doesn't work for him then the only other thing would be a full heart transplant, and we can't even think about that! Also, after his next stage operation his medication would change and he would live a restricted life with constant monitoring, which we really don't want for him. This had been the best news we've ever had about Christopher's health. The thought that Christopher may not need another major open heart operation was an absolute miracle. The old Justine in these circumstances would just eat and eat because of the stress and would have celebrated Christopher's good news with even more food, and then I would be feeling very tired and lethargic, stuffed on all the junk food. My favourite saying at the moment is: "Life is made up of luck. Good luck and bad luck!" When we eventually got all the results back from Christopher's tests there wasn't any miracle, Christopher needed to have his next surgery and very soon…

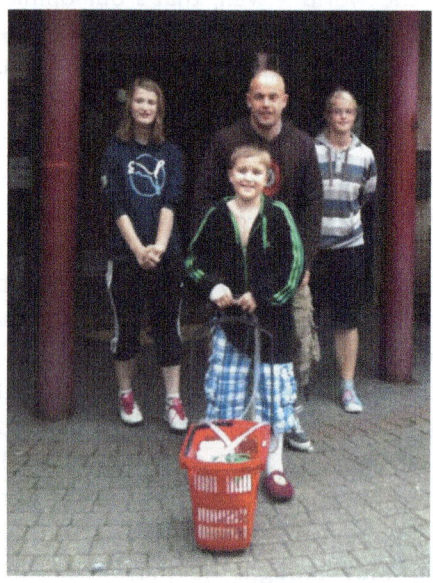

Christopher's operation 2011

Over the years, we've had to climb many mountains with our children but we've always managed it in the end. The life we lead as a family is a very, very close one filled with respect and love for one another. We bring our children up to appreciate every day, as you never know what is around the next corner. We also teach them tolerance and acceptance, as everyone isn't as lucky as they are and everybody in life is different, that perfection doesn't exist but happiness can be strived for. As long as they're happy and as healthy as they can be, our life is complete. Our children are the most important thing in our lives and we're so amazingly proud of all three of them; we never take them for granted.

At times, that has been one of the hardest things for me on this incredible journey: to understand and accept the way I used to eat and not give it any thought as to what I was doing to myself. The fact that, without thinking, I was doing so much damage to myself and my family. Health wise, I was solely responsible for eating myself into an early grave. I now find it very hard to understand how I could do that to myself and my family for all those wasted years.

What I have done is achievable for anyone with weight problems and I really want to get that point across to anyone who isn't happy with the way they are living their life and the issues they have with food. It's not easy, but it's also not that hard. You just have to have a little common sense and some willpower. I'm not special in the slightest, it's not been any harder or easier for me to do this. The only thing that sets me apart from the next person who gives up and doesn't make that change is that I wanted it more than them. I'm certain of that! My life in every way possible has changed. I don't think anything else in a person's life has the ability to change their whole being quite like a massive weight loss. I lived the last 20 years or so restricting myself because of ME! I was, in effect, living my life under my potential without realising it. Whatever problems life throws at you, life itself is pretty amazing. My motto now is: "Life is for the living". How true is that! Instead of feeding my habit of food these days, I've retrained my eating habits and now I can eat to live instead of living to eat. I find I don't want to comfort eat any more. If I'm troubled, these days I manage my stress in other ways, like going for a long walk with Nell, our family Westie, to clear my head. I can't tell you how I feel so much better from doing something like that instead of emptying the biscuit tin and feeling sick afterwards.

Millie and Christopher still have all their medical issues, there'll never be a miracle cure for what they have; in Christopher's case his operations are for palliative care and we all have to accept that and manage his health. Millie is a lovely, strong young lady, who I'm sure will live her life as only Millie knows how and attempt everything life throws at her with great determination and willpower as only Millie does best. She has found her niche in life through disability sports and competes up and down the country in her beloved discus. Millie's long-term goal is to get as good as she possibly can at it and maybe represent our country in it one day. Knowing our Millie, anything is possible! She attends a disability playground to podium events and was spotted in discus throwing, and was invited to train at Wigan Harriers by her coach, Bob Halliwell. We take her to Wigan twice a week. She's been all over the country this year competing in disability sports and she's aiming for the Paralympics in Rio 2016. She's ranked third in the country at discus at the moment and is certainly looking at bettering that over the next few months. She also wants to start competing in shot put.

Christopher is growing up to be a sensitive little man, I can just tell. Maybe we all spoil him, being the youngest and the only boy, but I really don't care – he's been through way too much and survived to tell the tale. I don't care that I spoil him – he deserves it! He'll also grow up knowing his limitations and he will do everything to his best ability, I'm pretty sure of that.

Christopher is limited because of his heart condition, but up until last season he played in goal for Longridge Town Under 11s. Since then his team has disbanded but he still goes along to the other team's training session every Tuesday night and really enjoys it. He's chosen to play in goal because then he can still be a member of the team but he doesn't need to run himself ragged. He still has to be careful of what he does because of the medication he's on and his heart condition; he can't keep up with his peers, but Christopher knows how much he can and can't do. He won a very special trophy at his football presentation – a new trophy in memory of his lovely trainer, Stephen Thackerely, who sadly passed away unexpectedly. Stephen was very understanding of Christopher's heart condition and would never push him too hard; they also shared their love for the same football team – Burnley FC. So for Christopher to get the Stephen Thackerely trophy was a massive achievement for him after everything he's been through. It was a very proud moment for us all when Lynne, Stephen's widow, presented our son with his trophy. Christopher has also been going to a local Stage Coach drama group and passed his LAMDA acting exams. He really enjoys it and is a proper little actor, and because it's not that challenging or tiring for him, unlike sports, I totally encourage it.

Alex, our Rapunzel… well, what can I say about Alex? She's the thread that stitches our family together. She's always supported and cared for us all and you can rely on her totally. She's very strong and loving and seems to do so well in everything she turns her hand to. She's very quiet and sensitive too. Alex stayed with me at Alder Hey Hospital when Christopher was born, and kept me sane for the whole nine weeks that we were there. She was only three at the time but she was so grown up for her age. Alex plays golf for Lancashire Girls after playing at our local golf club where she was spotted by the Lancashire Girls organisers and now plays all over the country and best of all, really, really enjoys it.

Every weekend the girls have competitions and Christopher has his drama. Life is never dull as we run from one activity to another and that's the reason we never go on holidays any more – we're way too busy with our kiddies and their activities, and we wouldn't have it any other way. The benefits they all get from their activities and hobbies are immeasurable.

All our children are very individual and all have a special role to play in our family; life truly wouldn't be the same without each and every one of them. Having my babies has been the biggest life experience for me, they have taught me so much and for that I'll always be grateful. I'm trying to set them a good example of how to live a healthy and happy lifestyle, and that in itself is so rewarding to see.

All three of our children are fighters, and I'm very proud to say they definitely get that gene from me!

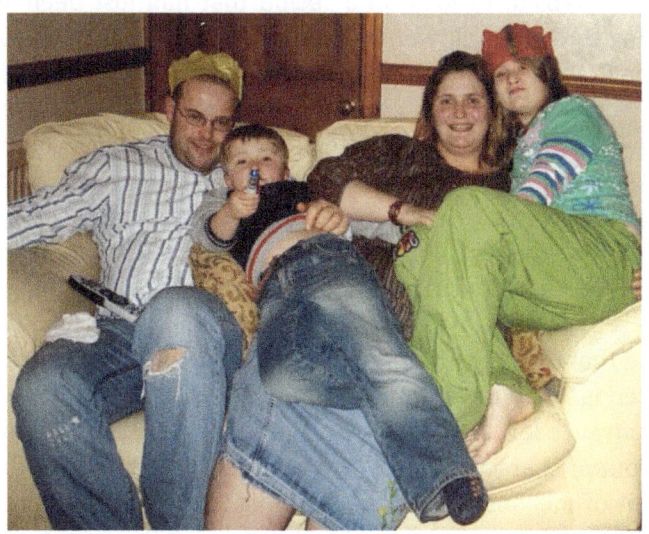

CHAPTER THREE

Michael Winner's Dining Stars

Believing in myself for the first time in 20 years – all because of my incredible weight loss! Going on to win a major television competition.

About eighteen months before this whole *Michael Winner's Dining Stars* experience started, I'd been watching *Come Dine With Me*; at that stage I hadn't lost any of my weight and certainly wasn't on any kind of diet/healthy living regime. I was probably at my heaviest in fact. I went on to the *CDWM* website to look up a recipe that had just been shown and whilst reading through their website information, I spotted an advert asking people in the Preston area to apply to go on the show. I still to this day don't know what possessed me, but I sent an email off to them explaining who I was and where I lived. Within minutes the phone rang. It was one of their researchers to interview me. I was then told someone else would probably ring me back at some stage.

I never really thought about it again as my life was full with the kids and everyday bedlam. Looking back, it seems such a weird thing for me to do because I'm really not into that kind of thing and had never done anything like that in my life before. Even though I love having a good dinner party for friends, I had never done anything in front of a camera. I was also suffering from such low self-esteem and confidence because of my size, so it was totally out of character for me to volunteer myself to want to do such a thing in front of millions of viewers. Within a few days, another researcher rang to agree a date to come and check my house over and bring a cameraman to film me for a demo tape.

I couldn't believe how nervous I was the day I opened my front door to the lovely producer Richard Bentley and his cameraman. I'm still very good friends with Richard and tell him regularly that he changed my life immeasurably and that I will always be grateful to him for that. Anyway, I spent that morning being interviewed and filmed for a place as one of the contestants on *CDWM*. We then had to wait for a few weeks as I was shortlisted and shortlisted again down to the last seven.

In the meantime it had been my birthday and to celebrate we had invited fourteen friends around for a meal. I cooked what I was going to cook if I got onto the show, as a bit of a trial run. I served home-made pate, followed by fillet steak, and pavlova for pudding. Just a few days after my birthday, Richard rang to say I hadn't made it but would I be their first reserve in case anyone dropped out, to which I agreed. It's weird in a way, because if I had have been chosen to go on *CDWM* then I definitely wouldn't have been used for the Michael Winner show. After that news from Richard I was a little disappointed but life went on and I never considered entering anything else, as I thought that kind of thing wasn't really my bag.

Fast forward eighteen months.

The date was the twenty-third of July 2009, and it's etched on my brain forever. The phone rang once more and the lovely Richard Bentley asked me whether I remembered him from the television programme *Come Dine With Me*. Of course I did – once you've met Richard you never forget him, he's pretty special. We chatted like old friends for a bit and I told him I'd lost 9 stone in weight since he had last seen me, which he found incredible. He went on to tell me about the show he was working on called *Michael Winner's Dining Star*s, and said he thought I'd be really suited to it and would I apply if he emailed through all the forms. He said it was going to be a great show and that, personally, he thought I had been too nice to go on *CDWM*. This new show wasn't going to be all about showing you up and making you out to be an idiot, and that I would really like it and enjoy the whole experience. I must say Richard and 12 Yard Productions sold it to me, it sounded great and very interesting. They said the winner would get to go to Michael's Kensington mansion and cook for all his A list friends, i.e. Simon Cowell, Piers Morgan, Phillip Green, John Cleese and maybe even Parky! The list was endless and very glitzy – who wouldn't want to win?

The next couple of months went by with Richard and others from 12 Yard Productions ringing me daily to ask me something or to tell me about changes etc. At this stage, I didn't even know if I had been picked to go on the show. In the same way as *CDWM*, a producer with a cameraman came to interview me and film me for the day. All the time in the back of my mind I told myself I wouldn't get picked, thousands had applied so why would they choose me, what made me so special? I was also right in the middle of changing my life and very busy turning it around for my family and me, so I really didn't give the show too much thought.

In the middle of September, Richard rang to say I had been chosen and they wanted to film Michael Winner having dinner at my house with my friends and family in the next two weeks. WOW! That's when the nerves set in and panic took over me. I couldn't sleep, and I was so nervous all the time I felt sick to the pit of my stomach. What had I done? What was I going to put my family through? I remember going for a long walk at four in the morning with Chris and Nell, telling Chris I really couldn't go through with it and that I was going to ring 12 Yard up and back out. It really did get that close – the pressure of not knowing how it was going to make my family and me look on primetime television was nearly too much for me to take. Did I need this in my life? Did I need to feel so nervous over something like this that I hadn't even really applied for?

I must have changed my mind at some point because I did go through with it and take part and thoroughly enjoyed the whole experience. It was something very few people ever got the chance to do and we did it, our little family from a small town called Longridge. We experienced and did some amazing once in a lifetime things over a period of about six months.

Exactly a week before Michael came to Longridge to have tea with us, a small crew came around to our house to film me and my family leading our everyday lives including walking the dog, playing together, baking and cooking, picking the children up from school and spending time together as a family. The series director on the show was Nic Guttridge. He's another person whom I've grown very fond of and am still in contact with. Nic will always be very special to me, just like Richard, and hold a place in my heart as he is the only man to ever have made my chocolate brownies ooze – and that's in his own words. He reminds me of the day I first made them when he was filming me. Funny little things like that stick in my mind when I look back on it all. The filming itself was pretty intense and very repetitive. Everything you did had to be done over and over again from many different angles. It was good to experience what goes on behind the camera and to see the things that, unless you work in that industry, you never get to see up close. Chris and I are so critical when we watch television now, especially reality shows.

The day arrived and Michael came for tea. I had to go shopping for all my ingredients and flowers beforehand. Friends in Longridge kept texting me all day saying they had just bumped into Michael Winner and that they'd seen the television crew in Berry Lane and at the Civic Hall. There was definitely a buzz around the place! If you were out and about in Longridge it would have been really hard for you to miss all the action going on as there was a very large number of crew and cameras, plus Winner barking his orders out to "Dinah", his PA, and the lovely Joan, his make-up artist, who is also still a friend of mine. Winner walked around Longridge, criticising my hometown and shouting at everyone. He then had lunch with all the crew in one of our local pubs and went on to make even more damaging comments about the food they were served, which hit all the local newspapers at the time and again when the programme was screened. Michael told me later that any publicity is good publicity, so they shouldn't have been too upset because he'd definitely given them that, good or bad.

Just before 6:00 p.m. our friends arrived to share the evening with the lovely Michael, followed by the arrival of all the television crew. I remember standing in the back garden with Nigel and Mary Morris, Alison and Steve

Wilkinson, and Chris and our children and being so nervous, as was everyone else as the pressure from the crew was immense. All the preparations that day had gone swimmingly, with no hiccups at all, but now terror was setting in as our little house became besieged by about thirty film crew. I didn't know most of the people walking around our home, it was the weirdest thing ever. Richard was there and Marie, my director, and the television crew who had been filming me all day. Then there was Winner's television crew and Nic Guttridge, his director, plus runners and "Dinah" and Joan and the lovely Mark Lesley, another director, and Matt, the boss from 12 Yard Productions. They'd blacked out the windows in the front room and moved all the furniture to the sides then filled it with their equipment and food and drink for themselves. I can laugh now, but at the time our lovely little "home" was trashed – literally. In our kitchen, they'd attached all these extra lights on the ceiling and they had brought loads of lamps for every room for extra lighting. There were wires and clips holding things up all over the place. They even removed doors! It really didn't look like our home any more, but to be honest I was having a panic attack and didn't really notice all the mess.

Just before 6:30 p.m. we were all ushered into the living room to wait for Michael to ring the doorbell and at that moment, just before he did, I went into meltdown and lost it for about five minutes. Marie, my director, ushered everyone apart from me and Chris out of the room and asked Chris to try to calm me down. I think Marie thought I was bottling it and I wouldn't go through with it, which had crossed my mind because I just wasn't in control of my space, my home and my family any more. I can't describe how frightening that felt. Everything calmed down and I drank a glass of champagne to calm my nerves, the doorbell rang and I was told to answer it!

As I walked into our hallway, Nic and Winner's crew filmed me, which I hadn't expected, and the bottom of my stomach dropped. I had to answer the door to this very frail, older than I had imagined, famous film director. I remembered when I was about eleven years old watching and being transfixed to all the *Death Wish* films, I loved them even though they were far too violent and sexual for my age. They came at a time in my life when my parents were going through severe marital problems and I was caught up in it all being the youngest child and the only one left at home to witness the full horror of what was going on. I used to stay up late and escape into a world of adult horror films and thrillers. So finally meeting the director and maker of these cult films that I watched at a very poignant time in my life, was incredibly exciting if not overwhelming for me.

When I opened the door to Michael Winner, I was struck with mental images of the Michael Winner that years prior had been in the papers for one thing or another. I had imagined a much younger and fitter man than the frail one standing right before me! I led him into our home by his arm and introduced him, one by one, to all our guests for the evening and our children. I sensed that Michael immediately warmed to me and my family, and since this time he has always been a very kind and generous family friend. He befriended me and the family on numerous occasions, always with humour and grace. I found him to be incredibly funny and very, very astute for his age. He's very honest, maybe a little too honest at times and it borders on rudeness, but I do admire the way he's not scared to speak his mind, and I wish at certain times in my life that I could have had the courage to do the same! I could sit all day listening to his very colourful stories about all the greats of our times, he really does have some amazing stories to tell, even if he does get a little too carried away with the name dropping.

Through the whole dinner party that evening Michael was very entertaining and funny and we all had a great time. In between courses, Michael would leave the table and go off into another room to talk into his Dictaphone and describe what he'd just eaten. While he was doing that the rest of the crew who weren't filming besieged my kitchen and ate all the leftovers from each course, even Dinah and Joan.

Then came the part of the meal everyone who watched the show remembers – Michael turned to me and asked about my weight loss. I told him I'd lost 10 stone so far. He rudely replied, "My dear, you must have been enormous – big isn't the word." I was shocked and paralysed by the thought of this going out in a primetime television slot for millions of viewers to see. All I could think about was changing the subject and at speed. Chris and some of my other guests had other ideas as they were very aggrieved about what Michael had just said to me and how he had said it. I grabbed Chris's knee under the table and squeezed it hard, to tell him not to carry on with this conversation. This part of the meal was by far the hardest bit for me after being under so much pressure to cook a meal and host the occasion. But I was very pleased at how everything turned out; for me I felt I couldn't have planned it any better.

We ate prawn cocktail for starters. I had laced my prawn sauce with a very big slug of vodka – I thought if I got him tipsy, I'd have a better chance of winning. For the main course we ate Beef Wellington with chunky chips and seasonal vegetables and thought it was perfect, as did the rest of the guests, but Michael thought a fillet of beef should never be wrapped in pastry. For pudding, I had made a strawberry pavlova with chocolate sauce. Michael didn't like this – he likes his meringues hard and brittle and mine are soft and chewy. Just before I served dessert, Michael was moaning that he'd heard around Longridge that I had a reputation for home-made baking and desserts and that I hadn't made him a cake! So as he went off to speak into his Dictaphone for the last time that evening, Chris turned to me and said, "Just make him something, something quick. I know you can knock a cake up." Still very flustered and frankly losing patience, I told him to shut up and not be so stupid – as you do when your husband suggests something daft. Minutes later, Nigel – one of the other guests – suggested the same thing and it suddenly seemed a good idea.

I dashed to my cupboards to see what I had. At that point, all I could think of was chocolate brownies – I have absolutely no idea where that one came from but all I can say looking back is that it was meant to be. Chocolate brownies have paved the way to huge changes in my career and I now bake for a living with my online business *Brownies by Justine Forrest*. I also make brownies and other delicious home-made cakes for coffee houses and other establishments around and about where I live.

But back to the evening... I proceeded to throw all the ingredients into a bowl for the brownies, and put them in the oven. They came out of the oven just as Michael arrived back to the table. I placed a warm chocolate brownie in front of him and suddenly he was in raptures. He said they were the best brownies he'd ever tasted! In his words, they were "historic beyond belief, a taste experience – perfection!" Wow!

We all said our goodbyes at the end of the evening not knowing if our paths would ever cross again, and as his driver pulled away in his very posh car, Michael turned to the cameraman and said, "Longridge – the land of the perfect brownie."

Five weeks went by after that memorable dinner party. Richard rang me nearly every day to run through arrangements and things and also about changes to the show. All the contestants were invited to London along with their dinner party guests and we were all to be put up in posh hotels for the weekend. The contestants were to visit Michael in an old cinema called the Coronet, in Notting Hill, where he would run through the entire evening he'd spent with us and tell us what he really thought about our hosting skills and food.

We were picked up by taxis at 5:00 a.m. to take us to Preston train station, then from there straight into London and onto the Coronet. At this point, it was very unorganised and the waiting around was unbearable. One of the other parties, the Wilkinsons, had brought along three of their youngest children but, because they weren't actually on the show, they had to stay in a Starbucks coffee house across from the Coronet for most of the afternoon until they had finished filming us.

One by one, we went through to meet Michael and were slaughtered by his cutting criticism of our evenings. This was done with military precision and none of the different dinner parties bumped into one another, as they were trying to keep us all apart until it came to the final stage of the competition – the two chosen finalists would have a cook-off, the winner being decided from that.

Michael was very cutting with his comments but he did like the fact my family and friends all stuck up for me and wouldn't be bullied by his comments. This stage seemed to go on forever; they kept stopping and starting the whole process. At the very end, Michael did his summing up of your evening and awarded you either one, two or three *Dining Stars*, in the form of a glass trophy, which you got to take home and keep. At a later date, I found out three of the contestants hadn't received any award, that they got no stars at all! Two of us – Peter and myself – got one star and Jane had two stars.

At my summing up, to my absolute astonishment, Michael broke down in tears and said he thought that I was heroic as a person and what he was doing was fickle in comparison. He said I had amazing friends and family. Heck… we were all crying! Filming that stage of the competition in the Coronet went on until one in the morning and Michael wasn't a happy bunny. I'm not surprised, they'd been filming for fifteen hours. We were lucky as we were the second out of six contestants to go through. We were now sworn to secrecy, as they didn't want the press finding out who'd won the show before it was screened. That was hard!

We had Friday to ourselves and together with the Wilkinsons, we hit the shops and went sightseeing. A fantastic day was had by all. We shopped in Harrods and went to see all the Christmas decorations – it was the middle of October and everywhere was trimmed for Christmas – WHICH I LOVE! Richard, the producer who was looking after me on the show, had promised to ring me at lunchtime that day to tell me if I had gone through to the next stage of the competition. If I had, I'd go to Winner's Kensington mansion the next day and meet the other two semi-finalists, and from there Michael would whittle it down again to the two he wanted in his final.

When Richard finally got hold of me on the phone I was pretty nervous, but I thought as I'd only got one star I was definitely going home. I was gobsmacked when Richard told me that I was going to Winner's house to meet him again! So, first thing on Saturday morning, Richard picked me up in a car to take me to Kensington. I was a little gutted as I said my goodbyes to my family and friends; up to this point they'd been with me through each stage and now I had to do this on my own.

My day consisted of being driven around London in a black cab, being interviewed over and over again whilst being in the same black cab and waiting around until Michael was ready for us. When we eventually got into Michael's palatial pad, all three semi-finalists were kept apart then taken into Michael's cinema room, which is situated in the basement of his house. The cinema itself has wall-to-wall framed photographs of incredible stars of the silver screen, people you only dream about, and my eyes must have been like saucers. The photos were signed with lovely messages to Michael. We were given a little time to get accustomed to the surroundings and waiting for us all was Nic Guttridge with his crew filming every move we made. Michael appeared and did a big speech, then we were given an opportunity to speak and convince him why we should be included in his final two. At the end of what seemed like hours, he chose Jane and me to go on to the next stage. I went back to our hotel in an absolute daze. I was so happy and Chris ordered the best champagne that the hotel had – that was when I got my taste for the bubbly stuff! We were leaving shortly after that to travel by train back home to Preston. At Euston, Steve nearly missed the train because he shot off to buy more champagne and snacks for us all for the journey home. In fact, the train had set off and he had to run down the platform and jump on it. I was quite intoxicated from the champagne at the hotel and wasn't aware of the drama he caused.

A week later and I was on my way back to London but this time on my own. This whole experience made me believe in myself more, and now found that I could do these things on my own. It had given me incredible self-belief and confidence for the first time in my life. Everything I had ever done in the past was with other people or for other people but this whole thing was about *me*. I found out I could do and achieve the things I wanted and I wasn't that useless after all! My weight loss had given me a confidence I never knew I had.

Once I got to London, I was met by the lovely Soph (as I call her). Sophie looked after me and chaperoned me to the hotel where I would be staying. Early next morning, I went down to breakfast and met up with Jane, the other half of Michael's final cut. Another film crew met us with another director, and we were taken to a warehouse somewhere in London that stocked all the film and TV props all the shows and films use. There were loads of things I recognised from the telly, like Jonathon Ross's sofa from his chat show. Little did I know that soon I would be sitting on it being interviewed by Jonathon himself, but that's another story.

Jane and I had to split up in the warehouse and were given two hours to choose every stick of furniture and soft furnishing that we thought we needed to kit a room out for our next dinner party. We had to pick everything from salt and pepper pots to glasses, pictures and even the table and chairs. That was so much fun! We got to run around a warehouse sticking Post-it notes onto everything we fancied. It seemed a weird stage in the competition, so that's why I think they never said anything about it on the show, as it didn't really make sense. Some of the favourite things I picked were a big stuffed sheep and a sack on cotton bales! We were told to have a theme for our room and mine was a *Northern Night In*. They didn't even explain that on the show. They even went to all the extra expense to hire and ship all that stuff to Cornwall for the final. Not to mention that it was a task in the competition still baffles me. I can remember one of the producers saying that he'd never worked on a show that had spent and wasted so much money on everything, especially at a time of recession. The show itself must have cost a small fortune to put together, and the things they wasted money on that never even got used was obscene. I know nothing about how that kind of stuff works but even I could see the massive wastage.

After choosing everything for our dinner parties, we both flew to Cornwall for three days, where we were taken to Polhawn Fort in Torpoint, which is situated on the western tip of Cornwall, to set up and start cooking for the final. Jane's party would be a lunchtime affair and mine in the evening. The day before the final, we both went shopping for all the ingredients that we needed and for everything else like flowers etc. We didn't do this together; we still had to be kept totally apart and were both filmed and followed by a crew all the time. I have to admit that I was very lonely and missed my family so much, I had never been apart from all of them for that long before. I was also very tired. It was all very intense being filmed all the time and the pressure to do your best, mixed in with all the travelling and waiting around, was very hard at times. When the final day arrived, we were both told that the winner's prize would be an all expenses paid short break with Michael. I thought I wasn't a particularly competitive person up until now, but the whole competition thing and meeting my rival, knowing I could cook as well as her, became all too much and I was determined to win. Jane was a really lovely person, but the pressure seemed to get to her and I don't think she could cope with it.

That final day felt like forever. Jane had been taken up to the fort very early that morning to prep for her meal and have her dinner party. I was so bored and nervous all day. Richard and I went out for a drive to kill time and we talked all afternoon as he tried to calm my nerves. Eventually, after what seemed like an eternity, Richard's phone rang and they wanted us both back at the fort so I could start prepping for my dinner party that night. I got stuck in. My meal was Spicy Butternut Squash Soup with home-made bread, Steak Pie with mash and vegetables, and for pudding Chocolate Heaven, which consisted of a slice of my famous chocolate fudge cake and a piece of my chocolate brownie served with fresh cream and some strawberries on the side. Michael sat at the head of table with Dinah, Joan and three hand-picked locals.

After it was over, I sat in the kitchen to reflect on how I thought it had all gone. One of the soundmen came in to eat up my left-over chocolate brownies. He casually said, "They didn't enjoy Jane's meal, most of it's been left in the fridge." I couldn't believe it! He went on to tell me that I'd definitely won. At around midnight, Jane and I were called through to see Michael again and to listen to his verdict on his whole meal experience. From the start of Michael's summing up, I thought it was going really well for me because for the first twenty minutes all Michael did was to criticise Jane's meal. I felt for Jane and held her hand for support. When Michael turned to talk to me all he said were nice things about my meal, apart from my mashed potatoes, which under pressure I had not put enough cream and butter into. I could tell that I was the winner straight away, so when Michael announced that the person who he wanted to cook for him and his celebrity friends was "Justine Forrest" it wasn't that much of a surprise, but in saying that, there's nothing quite like hearing the words that you've won or that you're a winner. I'd never won anything in my life before, so it was such a thrill! I celebrated with the crew and a few bottles of bubbly and can't remember going to bed that night.

The next day we arrived back in London and Richard took me to Euston. On the train home to Preston it all began to sink in and I started to get very excited, wondering where my short break with Michael would be? Afterwards I was to cook a final meal at Michael's home for him and his celebrity friends!

I spent the next few days washing, ironing, cleaning and cooking as I needed all my clothes packed again for my next trip, and I had to catch up with all my cleaning at home because it felt as if I had been away for months. Those days whizzed by and on Sunday, Richard was knocking at my front door again with his camera crew in tow. Back to lots of family filming and packing, then straight back to London. Once we arrived, Richard again chaperoned me to my hotel, the Hilton in Kensington, and informed me that I could have anything I wanted, no expense spared – I was the winner of the show and this was my treat!

Early the next morning, a car picked me up from reception and took me to a private airstrip somewhere in London, from there I met up with Nic and all the crew, and Michael and Dinah. We all boarded a private jet and I had no idea where we were going. Just before we landed at the other end of our journey I looked out of the window and there was a big sign that said Bruges. At that point, I broke down and cried because I would have loved to have shared the whole fantastic experience with Chris and the children – we'd never done anything as indulgent as this in our lives and I felt lost without them.

When you're with Michael Winner everything gets done at speed, everyone around him is subservient at all times, no one EVER answers back or disagrees with the man himself. I found that funny because out of all the time I spent with him, we actually had a good laugh and I think he appreciated the way I wasn't like that and I didn't lick his bottom or treat him any differently to anyone else that I'd met. I think that's maybe one of the reasons we're in contact with each other today; I'm probably one of the only people around him that treats him normally and I think he really likes that about me.

When we went through Customs we just walked through, I don't think Michael ever queues for anything, so that alone was a real experience. Michael and Dinah were driven away in a car while the rest of us had to wait for a mini bus for the drive to our hotel. We waited, we waited, and we waited. I think we waited for about an hour and a half in all. Someone from the production team in the office back in London had forgotten to order our transport... In the meantime, Michael and Dinah had arrived at the hotel and were waiting for us. Michael was not a happy bunny when we finally got there and the crew got a roasting. I, on the other hand, was enjoying the splendour of our hotel. My room was massive, a five star suite and the bathroom had two rooms in it.

Eventually Michael calmed down and we went for a walk. We were being filmed again and as Bruges has lots of visitors milling around, it caused a sensation – Michael Winner walking around with a camera crew! Everyone seemed to recognise him and stopped and stared at us all, it felt intimidating and very surreal. We then went for a boat ride together and were served champagne and strawberries; the bubbles went straight to my head as I'm not a great drinker. Bruges is absolutely magnificent and I loved every moment of my trip there, and I plan to take Chris and the children back to the very same hotel.

That night Michael and Dinah enjoyed their evening meal together and the rest of the production team and I went out for the evening. I really enjoyed this and needed to let my hair down. We all got on like a house on fire and Nic entertained us with stories of his social life. At the end of the night everyone went back to their hotel, and the other director Mark Lesley and I went out for a drink. We ended up getting completely lost and struggled to find the way back. At the hotel we met up with Dinah and Joan in the bar and it wasn't long before I was hitting the bubbles once again.

In the morning I got up really early and went for a long walk around

Bruges on my own. The sights were breath taking and at one point I broke down and sat on a bench crying because I so wanted my family with me to share it all. Just before lunch we all set off for the Gouden Harynck, a Michelin-starred restaurant not far from our hotel. Michael considered this to be one of the best in the world. I'd had my hair and make-up done and was taken into the kitchens to cook alongside the chef/owner Philippe Serruys, and his wife Maryke, who was front of house. I was in my element. Philippe and I exchanged tips on cooking and I'd like to think I gave him a few tips too that day. Later, Michael, Dinah, Joan and I had our lunch in a magnificent dining room. Michael and I had scallops with pureed chestnut, a second course of langoustines with cabbage and a delicious sauce. The main course was pan-fried partridge with wine, buckwheat on the side and chutney. For dessert, I ate a mango concoction and Michael had apple tart with vanilla cream.

It was now late afternoon and we all headed back to the private jet to return to London. The next day I shopped for Michael's chosen meal and went into all the shops he uses in Kensington. One of the shops was a very posh, organic health food shop and I got most of the ingredients there. I really enjoyed looking around at all the different foods they sold, some of which I'd never heard of before. I nearly fainted when the bill was added up and said out loud, "Oh My God, I don't spend that much on a week's shopping for the whole family!", it was so expensive. We finished all the filming for that day and Matt, the big boss from 12 Yard, thought it would be a nice idea for me to choose something to do at their expense. So accompanied by someone from 12 Yard Productions, I went to see *Wicked* in the West End. Chris and I had planned to take the children to watch it, so I was really looking forward to seeing it. I didn't really rate it much and found it a little boring, so at one of the intervals we went shopping instead and I bought a pair of the most fabulous purple UGG boots ever!

The next morning I was up very early once again and walked from my hotel to Harrods, where I bought Michael's birthday present, a wooden Jenga from their toy department and some very posh Harrods' chocolates. I paid an extortionate price for them to be wrapped professionally in their gift-wrapping department, ribbons and all. As I headed back to my hotel, I felt extremely sad because the whole experience was nearly over and some of the people I'd worked with over a period of four months would be going out of my life forever – I'm a very sentimental person at heart. A car came for me and I was taken to Michael's mansion, round the corner from my hotel in Kensington. Once there, I gave all the crew a hug before starting to prep for my meal that evening, but it seemed harder than before. I think it was because at this stage I was way too tired and homesick for my Chris,

Millie, Alex and Christopher and it was the end! And there was a camera crew everywhere. I don't think I have ever seen so many cameras and people in one place, you could hardly move and every time you did, you had to smile sweetly for the cameras and move people out of the way and make it look like you weren't frustrated; it was all very confusing.

In the middle of the afternoon, when I was about half way through my cooking, I was told who would be my celebrity guests for the night: Michael and Geraldine, Sir Roger Moore and Lady Moore, Christine Bleakley, Giorgio Locatelli, Andrew Neil and Kym Marsh. Well, I didn't want to sound ungrateful or anything, but I had been promised Simon Cowell and Piers Morgan! The menu Michael had chosen for me to make for his birthday dinner party was my spicy butternut squash soup with home-made crusty wholemeal buns, individual Lancashire hotpots served with sprouts tossed in butter with pancetta and my slow braised red cabbage with apple. For dessert it was always going to be my obligatory warm chocolate brownie with the very best vanilla ice-cream London had to offer. Everything was on schedule. At 7:30 p.m. all the guests arrived and were taken through to Michael's private cinema room to be served canapés, which I'd also made – mini pitta pizzas with capers, olives and fresh tuna. I was left in the kitchen to finish the cooking. Michael kept coming into the kitchen to talk to me between courses. I also had to serve at every course and tell the guests what they were eating. I had lovely assistants, a waiter and waitress, and managed exceedingly well with no hiccups.

At the end of the meal I was escorted out of the kitchen to change clothes and have my hair and make-up done by the lovely Joan and Dinah. Michael then called me through to the applause of all his celebrity guests. He made a big speech about me and my family and, to my complete surprise, my family appeared! I started crying, as I had no idea they'd been brought to London; all these arrangements had been made behind my back. My heart was filled with love as my family entered the room – all dressed to kill. I was *so* proud. I'd missed them so much it hurt. When everyone had stopped clapping, Sir Roger Moore awarded me with my ultimate *Dining Star Award* and Giorgio Locatelli kindly said that some professional chefs couldn't cook as well as I had, and that it was made even more special because it was all "cooked from the heart".

That night for my family and me will always hold a special place in our hearts. All the people who were involved in making it were a joy to meet and talk with, everyone was lovely and made it very special. After the filming had finished, we had time to go around and talk to everyone, Chris even got the chance to ask Christine to wear one of his beloved Burley Football Club t-shirts and have photos taken with her wearing it. He was in his element! Eventually all the guests left and Michael headed for his bed. We were taken back to our hotel where we got stuck into the finest champagne the hotel had to offer and proceeded to get very drunk.

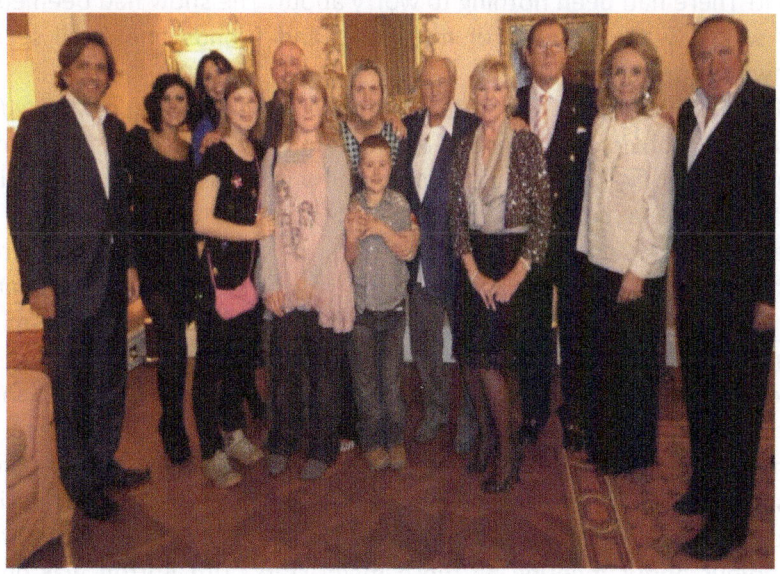

Next morning it was all over. We returned to our little lives once more after the excitement of the last few months. All that I had personally achieved was set firmly in our minds.

Fast forward to Christmas, then January, then February and things started to slowly build. Information was starting to come out about this new show *Michael Winner's Dining Stars*, and the buzz was growing. Michael rang me regularly and some of the production team also stayed in touch through phone calls and texts. Then one Saturday when we'd all just gone up to bed, one of my friends sent a text to say the show's trailer would be shown again, and it was! That was one of the most exciting things ever. From that moment on the trailer was played day in, day out. Every time I turned the telly on I was there dropping my prawn cocktails, it was funny. Then it hit the press and our phone was literally "HOT" every day.

Floods of magazines and newspapers wanted my story. I even had someone wanting to represent me and sell my story to the press for me, but I was still under contract to ITV and everything had to go through them first. In the end, I settled for a two-page spread in *Woman* magazine and numerous other press stories about my weight loss or how I made Michael Winner cry! This carried on for weeks and I started collecting all the cuttings from the stories – there were loads. The day of the show's airing arrived and I don't know how I got through that day, I was that excited. Since filming had begun I'd lost another 4 stone, so I was eager to see what I looked like on television. That night we went over to the Old Oak and had a party with all our friends and family whilst watching the show on the big screen. We all loved it! There had been nothing to worry about. The show had been edited really well. I was so proud of my family and friends and it all seemed worthwhile after the wait.

The next week, the ITV press office rang to ask if I'd go on *Harry Hill's TV Burps* and, obviously, I jumped at the chance because that's our family's favourite Saturday night show. Before I knew it, I was back on the train to London again and being put up in a posh hotel, all expenses paid. I was chaperoned everywhere. I was taken to the BBC Television Centre in Shepherds Bush, to spoof an interview for the Harry Hill show with Jonathon Ross. I had to go on Jonathan's show and he interviewed me in the middle of his television show *Friday Night With Jonathan Ross*. His show was pre-recorded, but because one of his guests that week was Johnny Depp and he couldn't make filming that night, they moved the schedule to the Wednesday instead. This fitted in perfectly with the Harry Hill filming on the Thursday. It was so much of a rush when we arrived at the television studios, terrible traffic made us late and there wasn't enough time for me to get nervous about meeting all these mega stars. Tim Burton was on the show along with Sir Andrew Lloyd Webber and 1980s singer, Sade. It was an incredible experience in the Green Room with them. I went through to the stage in front of Jonathan's packed audience while the act Four Poofs and a Piano sang "We're Gonna Make You a Star". After a short interview with Jonathan, I was then was ushered back to the Green Room, then back to my hotel for the night.

Next morning, after breakfast, Chris and the children arrived and we were all taken to the BBC Television Centre. I was taken into wardrobe, where they had bought me three new outfits, then through to the make-up department, where Harry was having his make-up done too. I gave him a big kiss and told him how much our children loved him. After chatting to me, Harry went into the studio to find Millie, Alex and Christopher, and for the very first time in their lives they were star struck, they were all completely speechless! Harry introduced us to all his crew and we rehearsed our song together, which took about twelve takes to get right. Later, we all watched what they had already filmed – about me and where I live in Longridge. We spent the next four hours watching Harry doing all the rehearsals for the evening show, which is filmed in front of a live audience. We had to rush back that night and couldn't stay to watch the show, but Harry invited us all back for his last show in the series and end of series wrap party. Wow!

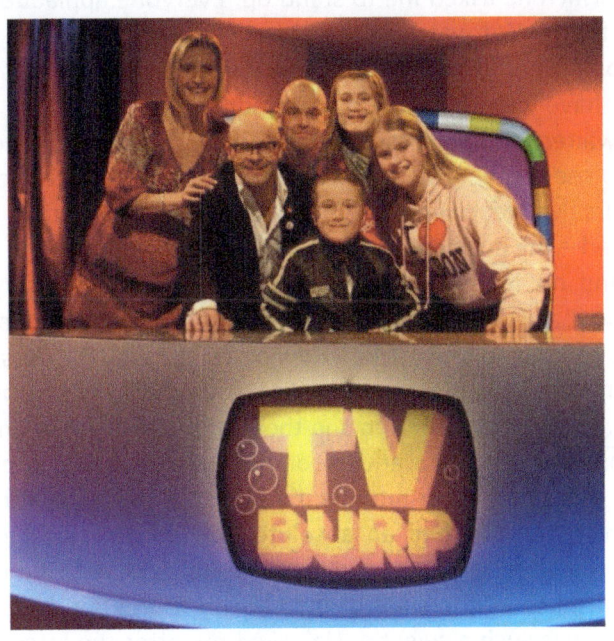

Two weeks later, Chris and I were on the train once again travelling back down to London to watch the Harry Hill show. We had our lunch at one of Michael's favourite restaurants, The Wolseley in Piccadilly. A few months before, all the family had eaten there with Michael, he'd treated us to Sunday lunch. This time, however, I couldn't get a booking, so I emailed the manager, Daniel Craig, who had looked after us with Michael. When we walked in to the restaurant, we found that Daniel had arranged champagne on arrival for us! The Wolseley is a beautiful place and the food fabulous. There were some very famous and recognisable people dining there that day and I sat alongside Melvin Bragg! We also bumped into Geraldine, Michael's fiancée, who was having lunch with one of her girlfriends. She came over to say hello to us all and have a brief chat. She wanted to know why I hadn't telephoned to tell them I was in London for a few days because Michael would have loved a catch-up with me.

After lunch, we headed back to our hotel and got ready for Harry Hill's show. When we reached the BBC Television Studios, we joined the queue to go through security. We were told that we'd gone to the wrong place and were shown to where we should be, which was through the front reception area of the main building. Once there, we were met by a guide and taken into Harry's Green Room, where there was food and drink laid on. A short time later we were shown through to our seats in the studio. Harry came onto the stage and announced that "Justine Forrest is in the audience tonight", to which he asked me to stand up. Everyone applauded, I thought it was very funny. We watched the show and afterwards we were taken backstage to another very large studio that had been kitted out for a party. There must have been at least two hundred people milling around the room, with waiters and waitresses offering fancy food and a free bar. Harry came over to see us, then the three other show writers started chatting and we found ourselves really enjoying the party. When it was time to leave we were surprised – the evening had flown by in a flash.

Harry and his team at Avalon were the highlight of everything I did during the Michael Winner experience. Everyone there treated us so well and made it all so enjoyable. The following week, the ITV press office rang again and arranged for me to go on *GMTV* with Michael to promote the show. Again, I travelled to London and they paid for me to stay in a very nice hotel. In those few weeks I went to London five times just to promote the show. So, in those few short months, I'd been back and forth from London at least eight times and had an absolute ball. When I went on *GMTV*, I experienced the Green Room again, make-up and refreshments before being introduced to all the stars of the show. I found Ben Shephard by far the nicest, he was such a sweetie. He asked me after the interview if I had brought my camera so someone could take some pictures of us, which we did. He was lovely.

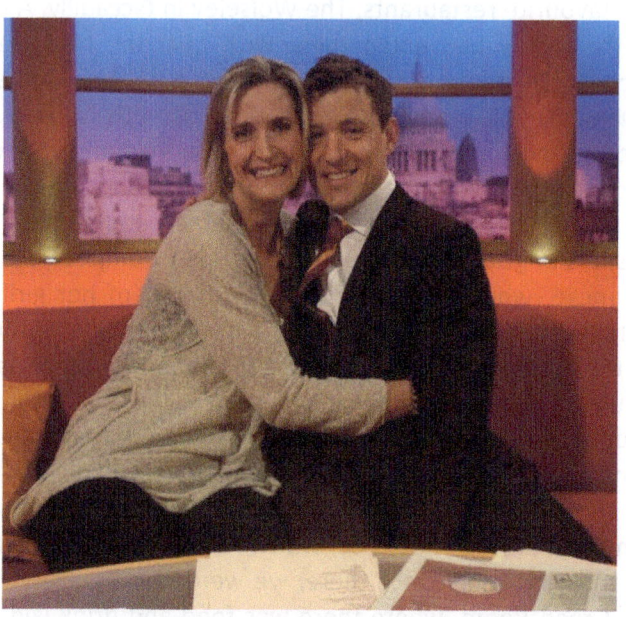

After the Michael Winner series had finally been shown on the telly and having won the series, I received lots of offers to do things. I attended a supermarket opening and cut the ribbon, and appeared on numerous radio shows, even having radio stations doing part of their shows from my house. I was in lots of newspapers and magazines and was recognised and asked for my autograph wherever I went. I spoke at charity evenings, opened a beer festival and was auctioned off to cook two dinner parties for a local charity. I can't remember half of the bizarre things I did, but everything was really exciting and we all enjoyed every moment of it with no regrets at all.

Who would have thought that that large lady from Longridge would do all this? I sometimes remember the promotional trailer for the show, which showed Michael and I crying whilst he was saying some very kind words to me. A little while after the show was screened, Michael appeared on *Piers Morgan's Life Stories*, during which they showed that clip. After he watched it again, Michael spoke to Piers about me and my family and his words were compassionate and kind.

* * *

I am forever grateful to Michael Winner for being instrumental in the whirlwind of change that occurred in my life.

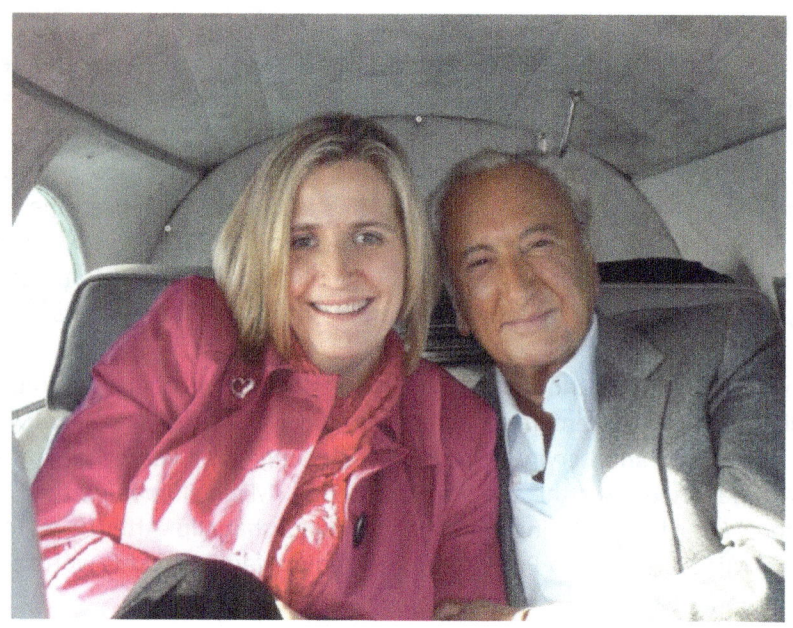

Since writing this chapter about *Michael Winner's Dining Stars* TV programme, Michael has sadly passed away at the age of 77. Michael had been diagnosed with terminal cancer in 2012 and was given eighteen months to live.

It was still quite a shock when BBC Radio Lancashire telephoned and broke the news. I sensed Michael was deteriorating fast, as contact over the previous two months had ceased. Since the show, Michael had kept in touch with me and would ring, tweet or email regularly to check on how we were all doing. He was very sweet to all of us and did a lot for me and my family. He paved the way for me to start my internet chocolate brownie company and he also encouraged me to start writing this book. I'm so sad that I didn't get the chance to give him a copy as he always sent me signed copies of his latest "scribblings."

RIP Michael Winner
You will be sadly missed by all of us here at the Forrest home. X

CHAPTER FOUR

Surgeries and Procedures

The surgery I've had since losing weight and why I've needed it.

A few years ago, there seemed to be a glut of television programmes about different surgical procedures to do with weight loss. I remember watching such a programme with Chris. The programme showed a young lady who'd had lost about 10 stone following a gastric band operation. She then had a further eight operations to remove excess skin caused by the effects of drastic weight loss.

I cringed as I watched the programme and said to Chris, "What's the point in losing all that weight if you end up looking worse after it and have to have surgery to correct all the hanging flesh." I thought that if I ever did lose a considerable amount of weight, I'd never be able to afford to pay for cosmetic surgery, so what was the point? Also, the thought of the procedures filled me with horror. Why would anyone put themselves through the risk of these operations just for cosmetic reasons? I believed that it was impossible to get rid of a vast amount of weight without surgery, which I could never afford, so what was the point of dieting?

Yet another excuse!

I gave up for yet another year because of the information I was getting from watching television. It would have made such a difference if, at any stage, I'd seen or read a positive story about someone, just like myself, who'd lost an incredible amount of weight on her own through exercise and healthy eating. If I'd seen before and after pictures of their body and its changes through healthy weight loss and could see how that person had gone on to have cosmetic surgery in a very positive and inspiring way, I think it would have made a difference to how I viewed the whole subject of dieting and surgery. It may well have been a turning point for me to rethink about how I was living my life and how I might achieve the same thing for myself. Everything that I saw had the opposite effect and made me give up completely. I watched several programmes about gastric bands and stomach bypass operations and considered them to be my only option. I never thought it was possible to do what I have done on my own. That's why I'm so passionate about spreading the word and trying to inspire others who want to help themselves to do something about it. The television programmes on those surgical interventions made me mad back then, now they infuriate me! They put me off those procedures completely.

I don't think a gastric band or a stomach bypass operation is the way forward or an easy option. I think the medical profession offers them too easily, instead of trying to educate people on good food and exercise and addressing the real issues that cause overeating; they offer expensive surgical procedures and not enough information. It's not the way forward for this obesity epidemic nor a miracle cure. Support and advice and help with getting motivated should be more available. A gastric band or bypass isn't a magic wand and you still have to eat less and exercise more. In some cases, the patient even has to lose a considerable amount of weight *before* their surgery because operating on someone so huge creates high risk.

I once heard that if you asked your doctor, you could get a reduced subscription to join a local council-run gym, so I asked my doctor and was told I could only get one if I was monitored by the nurse regularly. At that point I had only lost a couple of stone and was still highly embarrassed about being overweight and wouldn't let anyone near me with weighing scales, so that option was totally out the window for me. I think it's ludicrous that this type of activity is not available, free of charge, to encourage you to lose weight when you are seriously obese, as I was. The government should encourage gym membership. Investment now would save the NHS long term on weight related medical conditions.

An eating addiction is so hard to conquer and maintain. With other addictions you have to quit, with food you still have to eat, and for me that makes food addictions the hardest and most complicated of all addictions to master. To me, there are simple solutions for people who want to help themselves. Not everyone will succeed, but I truly believe if it's dealt with properly and all the information and help is out there, we can all do it. It's not always about how you look or being that size 12 – the real key is being healthy and living a long and healthy life. Educating the next generation on how to live a healthier lifestyle and make the right choices for themselves is *so* important. We need to start at ground level and get kids involved with healthy, tasty cooking and doing more physical activities in schools. There should be no excuse for any child not being able to exercise, in or out of school. I have two children with medical needs and disabilities; they experience exercise and sport in different ways, tailored to their needs. Everyone knows the importance of staying in shape. It doesn't have to mean a kick ass workout at the gym either – walking is such an underestimated exercise. With all the knowledge we hold about fitness and diet, we should all by now know the basics and be able to put them into practice.

But back to my surgeries...

When I had lost 6 stone, I went to my doctor to ask for information about skin removal after weight loss. He told me to come back when I was down to the size I wanted to be. So about nine months later I went back. My doctor was amazed that I had lost another 8 stone and was now thinking about cosmetic surgery to remove excess skin around my stomach. He said he would send me to our local hospital for a consultation about all the procedures. Five weeks later, I received my appointment to see my plastic surgeon, Dr Laitung. I remember the appointment so well.

First, I was weighed and measured by a nurse before being taken through to a side room and told to undress, put on a gown, and wait. Chris and I sat there, not knowing what to expect. Eventually Dr Laitung came in and he asked me to remove my gown. Agh! I don't know who I felt sorrier for, him or me! He looked through my hospital notes and asked, "Have you had a gastric band?" to which I proudly told him that I'd lost the weight all by myself. He was astonished and told me that people don't lose that much weight without having other surgery first.

He proceeded to lift up the excess skin from around my stomach and chest area and explained about the operation he was planning, called an abdominoplasty – a tummy tuck. This is a little bit different from the usual tummy tuck and starts between the breasts and goes down and across your tummy in a fleur-de-lys pattern. Dr Laitung then moved around my body and discussed a breast uplift (mastopexy) to remove all of the loose skin from around the breasts and to lift them. My breasts had shrunk so much and were now low, empty sacks of skin. Then a thigh and buttock lift (thighplasty). I'd lost so much weight from my legs and bum and was left with a lot of loose skin there. No amount of exercise and healthy eating would make it disappear, I needed the surgery. Finally, he would do an arm lift, to remove all the loose skin from my arms and get rid of the bingo wings. Well, I didn't know whether to be very grateful or very hacked off! I'd not noticed how terrible I looked naked until it was all pointed out to me by the lovely Dr Laitung. I asked him how many more consultations I'd need before my operation. He told me that the next time we'd meet would be in hospital, in seven weeks' time. Chris and I froze. I didn't want to sound ungrateful as I was having this all done on the NHS, but I couldn't have it done that soon as I was due to promote *Michael Winner's Dining Stars*. I explained this to Dr Laitung. He was very pleased for me and kept saying I must be a celebrity! We agreed to postpone my operation and they would recall me in three months, which was excellent because I got calls from *GMTV* and *Harry Hill's TV Burps* and the *Jonathon Ross Show*, also numerous other radio shows, magazines and newspapers and appeared on them all.

The day before my operation I took lots of photos of my tummy as a reminder. Up until that point I was very upbeat about the operation and hadn't given it much thought. I certainly hadn't thought through the enormity of it all. My friend Alison took me to hospital as Chris was working. I was confident that I could handle it all on my own. This time, though, it was completely different – I didn't have any children with me. With the children it's always a hospital trip for something really important, an operation that they need, not a frivolous procedure like a tummy tuck. In Christopher's case, operations were to keep him alive. I suddenly realised that I knew nothing about this operation, not even how long I was going to be in theatre or how long I was going stay in hospital. Was I being totally selfish by putting myself and my family through all this with all its risks just for cosmetic reasons? I can't tell you how many times I nearly walked out that day, and the next.

On the ward a nurse escorted me into a bay, settled me in and filled out my admission forms. To my horror there were three other ladies on the same bay, all of whom were very old and frail, and the smell made me feel very sick. As soon as the nurse left I cried, feeling very sorry for myself. Later when Chris arrived, some of the nurses noticed how upset I was and asked if I wanted to move to another bay to be on my own, which I did. Slowly I began to cheer up. I like to be on my own with my own space and this actually had an impact on my recovery – when my noisy children came to visit me we could just be normal and weren't annoying anyone else.

The morning of my operation came. Dr Laitung appeared with his registrar to mark my stomach with a black pen. I stood in my birthday suit and heard Dr Laitung tell everyone, "This is Justine, she's a celebrity chef." I was so embarrassed! He told them about the television show I'd won and went into raptures over my famous brownies (I'd taken two boxes with me). I remember lying in the anaesthetist's room waiting to go to sleep, listening to different doctors and nurses ask where they could buy the brownies and that they tasted amazing!

I was in hospital for nine days after my tummy tuck operation. There was a complication with one of the drains and the stay felt like forever. When I got home from hospital, it was a week until my fortieth birthday and a group of friends had organised a weekend away, camping in the Lake District. I needed to be in a hotel as I was recovering from the operation, I couldn't sleep on a blow-up bed, and I was pretty much out of it from medication so I didn't even get to toast my birthday.

Three months later I went back to Dr Laitung and had my tummy checked over. He looked at the scars and was a little disappointed about how it had healed and spoke about having the scaring removed at a later date. I was quite shocked – to me it looks fabulous! A million times better than it did before. We discussed the next operation, the thighplasty to remove the loose skin from my thighs and buttocks. There would be scars but I wasn't worried. After this would come the breast lift and last of all, the arm lifts so I would no longer have huge bingo wings!

All of these operations are the drawbacks of having lost a tremendous amount of weight. I'm very open about the fact I've been on this journey on my own, without the help of a gastric band/stomach bypass operation or any other procedures, and I'm also quite open about all the cosmetic surgery I've undergone or am undergoing – caused by me being morbidly obese. I'd really love this to be a lesson to anyone who reads this book – to learn from my mistakes. For all the years I over-ate and stopped caring about myself, for me this journey isn't just about changing my lifestyle, getting fit and losing the weight, it is also about having to undergo major surgery just because I stopped caring and comfort ate my way to obesity.

Since beginning this book I've undergone another skin removal procedure and have had excess skin removed from the inside of my thighs. This was straightforward – I went in on the Monday before Easter, had the op on the Tuesday and came back from theatre a couple of hours later with drains in both legs, staying in hospital until Friday. It was Good Friday, and a very *good* Friday for me as I was discharged and went home. The post-op on this was the hardest, so much worse than anything I'd been through with surgery before. I struggled to walk and sleeping was extremely uncomfortable. Sitting on the loo was out of the question and it was impossible to have a bowel movement standing up. I also learnt to pee like a man! The pain was excruciating when I sat down because I had been stitched from my knees right up into my groin. Ouch!

That was only half the problem. Every week for about a month, I had a series of infections in my wounds and was back on the ward needing intravenous antibiotics, amongst other treatments. I was in hospital for Millie's fifteenth birthday and it was awful. I can't describe how I felt at not being there for her, for the first time in her life. I was very poorly, the infection was bad and my temperature was just short of 40 degrees. I'd lots of orders waiting to go out for my online business, and Chris had to pack up and deliver them all. It's such a strain when you're trying to juggle your life around these extra problems. Eventually my scaring started to heal but unfortunately my right foot has remained swollen. A year later and there's no change and I can't wear heels. My surgeon says it's poor circulation and it might come back a little in time. That's the price you pay and the price you must way up before having any surgery.

My most recent achievement on my journey is that Chris and I ran the London Marathon and didn't walk or stop once! My right foot managed the distance, so I can cope with it.

On the whole I'm pleased with my surgeries so far. My stomach is amazing and I would say it's a must for anyone who has lost a massive amount of weight and wants to get on with their life. If I hadn't had surgery to remove the skin from that area, I most definitely wouldn't be running now, as it was impossible to run with that much skin swinging around and it was also very painful. The skin removal on my thighs, to me, looks amazing too; it's far from perfect and is uneven in places, but what is "perfect"? With all my post-op complications, I'm still trying to decide whether the thighplasty was genuinely worth it. I would say that it is, but I went through a massive amount of pain and discomfort.

With all the surgery my family has endured, you'd think we would be pros at it by now. Unfortunately, every time one of my babies has an op, I struggle to cope and look for comfort in food – any food just as long as I can chew and swallow it. This situation happened again recently as Christopher underwent his third major open heart surgery at Alder Hey Children's Hospital. This was the first time either Millie or Christopher has had surgery since I've lost my weight. As well as trying to cope with what we were all going through, I was very conscious that this was going to be another personal test for me. I didn't really know how to cope with my comfort eating again. I knew it would raise its ugly head while I was nursing my son back to health. Just being away from home and family life, having to cope with all this and trying not to eat junk food and snack – my way of escaping from this very lonely and sad situation we were all in – could I cope? Had I changed the way I looked at and controlled my eating habits enough for me to not look upon food as a way for me to feel better, if only for that minute I'm eating it?

It was a huge personal test for me. I watched Christopher fight for his life for six weeks. Every week he would seem to get a little better then wham bam some other complication would raise its horrible head and he'd need another emergency operation. Six times he headed back to theatre, each time the situation seemed worse than the one before. It was heartbreaking, and even now brings tears to my eyes to think about what he went through. I really don't know how we all coped. It was the saddest time of our lives. It got to the point even some of the nurses would cry along with me; for those six weeks nothing seemed to go right. Everyone back home who knew us was amazing with their love and support. We had supportive messages through Facebook and cards and presents from all over the world which was incredible and helped immensely. The chocolate supply for Christopher never stopped and, you've guessed it, was mainly eaten by me. That and masses of junk food from the hospital canteen. I did have facilities to cook over at Ronald McDonald House, where I was staying, but because of my nature, whenever one of us is in hospital, I can't bring myself to leave their bedside for long, so the thought of cooking a meal for myself wasn't an option, although I would boil up a little pasta from time to time when money got tight and I didn't have any for a canteen meal. Friends used to send things in with Chris, so that always helped too.

I'd recently been approached, through my agent, to front a campaign for the charity Ronald McDonald House for their new house being built at Manchester Children's Hospital. Through the charity, Chris and I got places in the Great North Run and the London Marathon. We must have been mad because neither of us had run since school, and said yes before we'd even attempted to do any running. I'd gone to the hospital with Christopher with good intentions but I had swollen legs and feet from being three months post op. I even took my running stuff into hospital with me, but as the days turned into weeks and everything started to go pear shaped, I just couldn't drag myself away from my poorly son. So at that stage and after trolley loads of comfort chocolate and snacks I decided to just eat what I wanted as I couldn't cope with thinking about myself and concentrate on eating healthy and maintaining my new body weight.

Eventually, and very slowly, Christopher started to get better and was discharged. As we drove away from the hospital Chris pulled into a Sainsbury's in Liverpool and we bought our "last supper", which consisted of some nice seafood to start with, then a lovely bit of rib-eye steak and veggies all to be cooked by Chef (me) at home. It was lovely.

Oddly, the minute we got home I knew this was going to be my last supper and that I was going to be on it again like sonic until I lost the weight I knew I had put on through sitting at Christopher's bedside for six solid weeks with no exercise. It wasn't about what I was eating, it was the lack of exercise too. I hadn't really done much back at the gym after my operations than I was in hospital again. All in all, I didn't exercise for about four and a half months. Not even a walk or two either.

At home, I put our scales in the loft again – just as I had done all those years ago when I started losing weight. I wasn't even tempted to check my weight. I knew that if I did, it would depress me and make it even harder for me to stay focussed and there would be a chance that, instead of being determined to lose the weight I had put on in hospital, I might be so depressed that I could just put on even more and gain most of my weight back.

So first thing the next morning, I was up and ready to start my training for the Great North Run. We set off jogging around Longridge. We only had two and a half weeks until our run and I'd never run a single mile in my adult life; in fact a couple of years before I couldn't even walk for ten minutes never mind run! Two and a half weeks later we ran without stopping or walking the whole 13.2 miles in the GNR and we raised nearly £2,000 for RMHC. Every step of the way was inspired by what our son

Christopher had just been through. It felt amazing to be able to give a little back, for all the love and support that had been given to us on so many occasions over the last eleven years of our son's life. I would always recommend having a goal you can work to and achieve, it keeps you on track and focussed. By Christmas that same year, I was back in my jeans and felt fit and healthy once more.

So the motto of this story is: *Don't beat yourself up because you can't be good all the time.* It's all about knowing when to bring it back and balance the books. Life is way too short to live any moment with regrets.

There is always tomorrow.

Since then, Chris and I have run the London Marathon without stopping or walking – a massive personal achievement for us. You can achieve anything you put your mind too, all you've got to do is want it enough!

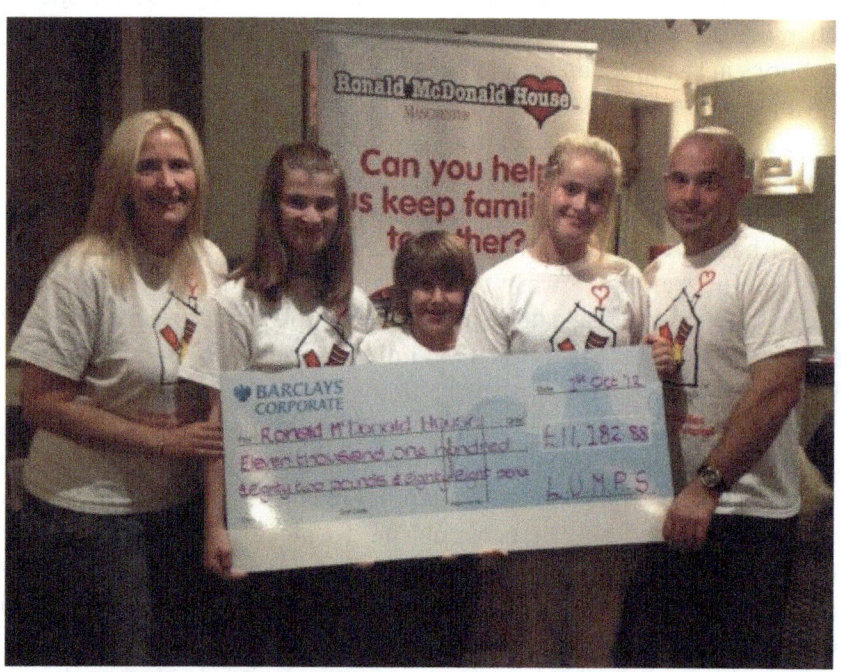

CHAPTER FIVE

Exercise!

The different types of exercise I've tried and incorporated into my daily routine, including descriptions and clarification from qualified gym instructors.

From day one, I knew I had to do it. For me, exercise has always been very motivational. It clears my head and releases endorphins, which makes me feel fantastic. These days I maintain my weight through exercise. I can have treats because I know I'm working them off and keeping myself fit, and life would be so boring without the odd treat or two.

In the beginning, I injected exercise that I enjoyed doing into my everyday routine and used it to keep me on the straight and narrow. It was so hard for me to even walk a short distance in the beginning, and the thought of putting all that effort in and then eating too much the rest of the day made me stay focussed on the changes I wanted to make to myself and my lifestyle.

At first, I started by walking near my home. I took our little Westie dog, Nell, with me for company. I went out walking for ten minutes each day and believe me, that was hard! In those days, my clothes consisted of two huge denim skirts, size 32 – I couldn't get anything else to fit me – and wore baggy t-shirts and cardigans on top. In warm weather, I took a large tub of talcum powder with me and applied this onto my legs every few yards, as they would rub together badly and leave friction sores if I didn't. In time it got easier, and I gradually built up stamina to be able to walk for an hour, twice a day. Once in the morning when I'd dropped the children off at school, then an hour in the evening with Chris. We still try to get a walk in as often as we can – we love the time we spend together walking around Longridge, discussing the day's events.

For the first year, walking was the only exercise I did. I lost 10 stone by doing this combined with eating healthily. *IT CAN BE DONE!* You don't need to spend a fortune on a gym pass or fancy training equipment, all you need is a pair of comfy shoes and you're off. As long as it gets you a little out of breath and sweaty, it's working. Nell is now the fittest dog in Longridge too! We'd bought Nell for Alex's tenth birthday; she'd always wanted a little dog and we had friends that bred West Highland terriers. Nell was one of the instigators in me getting healthy and fit. We'd had her for nine months before I started to walk her, before this Nell never got out. I felt really bad about this and wanted to change it, so I led by example, and now Chris and Alex and I can be seen with our Nell in and around Longridge daily. Nell also has a large selection of outfits to fit every occasion and is ready for all weathers.

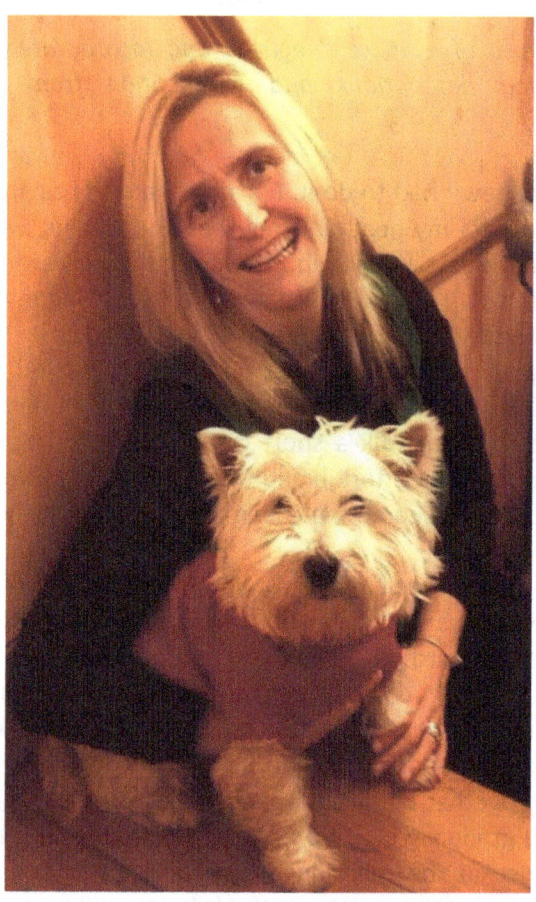

After a year of walking and getting much fitter, I found myself wanting to push on and try other exercise, so I joined our local gym: Kingfisher. My life has never been the same since. I have a handful of pinnacle times in life and joining my gym is definitely one of them, as it has changed my life in every way – from making lots of new and wonderful friends to learning so much more about my health and body.

I love everything at the gym, all the classes, the socializing and the people there. At the beginning of my journey, Chris had suggested I join Kingfisher as he had been a member for some time and really enjoyed it, but because I was morbidly obese and had absolutely no confidence in myself, the thought was far too frightening! I imagined gyms being full of very fit, slim people who would stop and stare at me in horror. Of course, it's not like that at all. Everyone is warm and welcoming and non-judgemental. I am very lucky that I found such a good place to exercise in, and if you are considering joining a gym, search around until you find a place that feels comfortable to you.

There are personal trainers at Kingfisher and they have become good friends of mine. They support, advise and help, nothing is ever too much trouble for them. Through their encouragement and guidance, I have gradually understood so much more about exercise and myself. In the section to follow, I've written about the exercises I've tried and tested. You could experiment and try something different yourself. What works for me isn't necessarily going to work for you, but you won't know unless you try it!

Remember: *It is important to discuss any activity programme with your doctor before you begin.*

ZUMBA

Longridge has been gripped by Zumba mania in the last few years thanks to our very own Leah Townsend, who works at my gym. She's been on the course and has the certificate to prove it. She is absolutely amazing. There aren't many women who can move their hips like she can! Sadly, I am definitely not one of them. I try very hard though and want to persevere with Zumba because once you get into it, it's a great laugh and so much fun.

I hated Zumba at first, mainly because I was so bad at it and felt very self-conscious doing it. Then I had an idea – take Chris with me and that would make me look much better. Wrong! Chris is great at it and makes me look even worse. Serves me right! But I persevered with Zumba and now I love it. I just had to get over that group thing, AGAIN! The whole point of Zumba is to let your hair down and have a good laugh, it's not serious, everyone just does their own thing.

Leah has graciously written a description of Zumba for us, so you can understand what it's all about.

Zumba by Leah Townsend

Zumba is a fun, dance based fitness class that fuses hypnotic Latin rhythms and easy-to-follow moves to create a one-of-a-kind fitness programme that will blow you away. Most people hate working out but Zumba makes you want to do it, love working out and you get hooked. Let's face it, working out can be healthy, rewarding and beneficial. Working out can be a lot of things, but it's never been known to be an exhilarating experience... UNTIL NOW! Zumba fanatics achieve long-term benefits while experiencing an absolute blast in one exciting hour of calorie-burning, body-energizing, awe-inspiring movements meant to engage and captivate you for life. Zumba routines feature interval training sessions where fast and slow rhythms and resistance training are combined to tone and sculpt your body whilst burning fat. Add some Latin flavour and international zest into the mix and you've got a Zumba class! In past years, the Zumba programme has become nothing short of a revolution, spreading like wildfire and positioning itself as the single most influential movement in the industry of fitness.

Zumba can be enjoyed by men and women, but is most predominately attended by women, despite the fact that the creator is male. Zumba is different to many other fitness classes, for example aerobics. In an aerobics class it is essential to follow exactly what the instructor is doing; with Zumba, as long as the movement is safe then the instructor allows you to put your own style and flavour into the dance, therefore the individual can enjoy the workout rather than concentrating on what everyone else is thinking. This influences people to join Zumba because they don't feel intimidated and pressured into keeping up with everyone else. The number of calories burned depends on the individual, how much they put into it, how much exercise they are used to doing etc, but on average people burn 500–600 calories per hour session.

In a nutshell, Zumba is all about having fun and working out without even realising it. Most people come out of a class dripping with sweat and really feeling that they have achieved something, but at the same time not having to look at the clock wondering how much longer they have to go.

Leah Townsend – *Manager of Kingfisher Gym Longridge*
Dance Instructor, Level 2 Gym Instructor, Personal Trainer, Qualified Exercise to Music Instructor, Circuit Training Qualifications, Spin Qualifications, Zumba – Basics 1 and 2, Zumba Gold, Zumba Training, Zumbatomic, Zumba Aqua, Kettlebell Qualifications

So that was Zumba. Now onto another passion of mine – Spinning!

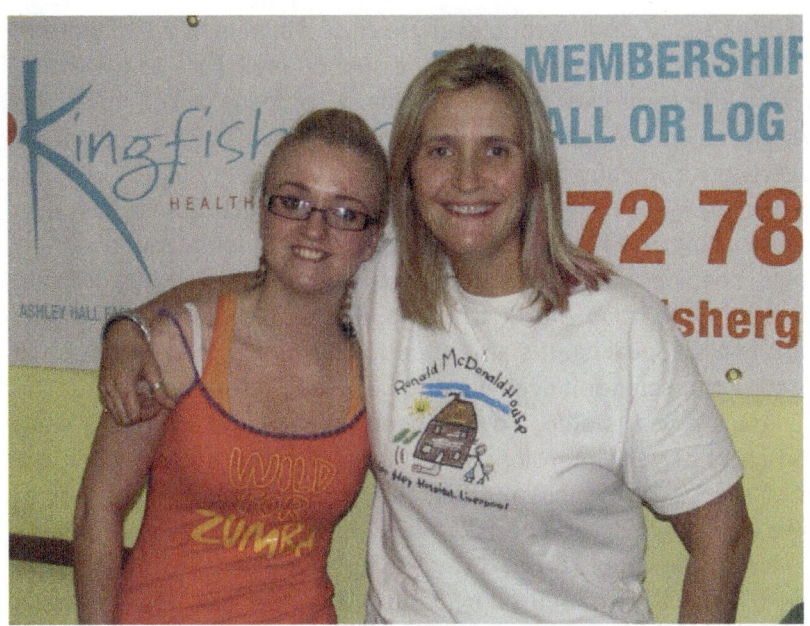

With Leah Townsend Zumbathon November 2011

SPINNING

I love spinning. It was the very first group thing I tried at my gym and now I'm hooked, as they say. I go to spinning classes five or six times a week, I enjoy it that much. Doing it in a group setting really pushes you on and doesn't give you that element of giving up. You can make it as hard or as easy as you like, you're not in competition with anyone else. All you need for this class is a water bottle, towel, trainers and gym clothes, you don't need anything fancy, so don't waste your money. It's a giggle at times, especially at the start when you're all warming up and when it's finished and you're cooling down. You feel so good about sweating it out and burning all those extra calories off, it really does lighten your mood and make you feel fresh for the whole day. Everyone should have a go at spinning; I know it's not for everyone but I think you should at least give it a go – you really don't know what you're missing until you've tried it!

Our lovely instructor, Darren, has helped me out and written a description of spinning, so you can understand the ins and outs of it.

Spinning by Darren Salmon

Why spinning? What is spinning? Two of the most commonly asked questions. It's indoor cycling, to give it its real name, and it became popular in the 1980s as a new cardio group exercise class. Spinning is a cycling term used by most cyclists – "I'm going out for a spin on my bike"– as the action of pedalling a bike looks like you are spinning. A company picked up on this and now they own the name, so not everyone can go spinning, it all depends on which company trained the instructor.

Why cycling indoors? Well, if you're a cyclist, short intense sessions, 30–40 minutes long, will help improve your cadence, or leg speed, on either flats or hills. Keeping a steady pace on a bike outdoors is always difficult, especially when the road starts to climb. For non-cyclists, low impact exercise is always appealing. It's also good for beginners too. Do you need any bike skills? No. You don't even need to be able to balance on a bike. The bikes you use are very stable. Do you need to use hand signals to warn other road users of your intensions? No. Maybe the odd one or two in the direction of the instructor, but nothing too technical! Do you get wet or wind blown? No. Every day is a perfect biking day indoors. Do you ever get a puncture? No. Some people do go away feeling a little deflated though. Has anyone been hit by a car or abused by a motorist whose only touch of fresh air is watching Emmerdale? No. So if you have fit people and non-fit people in a room doing the same thing, how do they all benefit? No one wants to sit next to a budding Bradley Wiggins or Victoria Pendleton, it can be very intimidating and off putting. The instructor sets the pace, or cadence, and everyone follows the pace after a 5–10 minute warm up. If, for instance, the task is set where it's a fast road, the pace will be to a fast punchy beat of music. What makes it difficult is the tension put on the wheel by you, by turning a round lever under your handlebars. No one knows how much tension is on your bike, only you; if it's hard work for you then it's enough. No one checks, it's entirely up to you. If you cheat, there is no point really, it's only you who is cheating yourself. If your fitness level is not very high, you might need a rest to begin with. Every journey starts with a single step forward. If you want results, you have to put the effort in, and the pain is usually worth the gain in the end. It is one of the few classes where everyone looks to be doing the same but in the end, results can be totally different.

The tension on your bike to simulate a hill climb is a good way for people to improve their leg strength at a slow pace. Working the pedals uses big muscle groups, quads and hamstrings and it is a great challenge. Seated and standing climbs are as hard or as easy as you make them because, as with on the flat, it's your hill and your tension.

The Ribble Valley, where I live, is a good place to test your new-found cycling skills. Flat roads and hilly climbs are plentiful; just try to avoid people with flat caps and whippets going to the dark satanic mills of yester year.

Some instructors use press ups and dips, even lunges on the bike – personally it's not for me, as I have never seen anyone do them on The Tour. To me, cycling is all about legs, and with respect to other people's preferences, it's up to each instructor as to what they do, so it's always worth checking their class out first. Each instructor plays a big part in indoor cycling, they pick the music you're doing it to and they motivate and inspire you. The majority of instructors aren't people who have just jumped off the cover of a health magazine or an aerobics television episode. If they look reasonably fit, there is a good chance their workout will work for you because, at the end of the day, we're all looking for the same end result: to look good and be as healthy as we can. Look for an instructor that is knowledgeable about a bike set-up. If the bike set-up is wrong, for instance the seat height or handlebar distance, then your 45 minute spinning class could feel uncomfortable and with a big chance of an injury to your knees, neck or back. You need an instructor who will help you on your fitness journey in a safe and effective manner. Any idiot can urge you on, but not everyone can motivate you into coming back and building your confidence and help you make a better body to live in. Not many people want to be shouted at by some self-opinionated, loud mouth instructor hell bent on improving their own fitness and showing off how fit they are.

What do you need? Water, a towel to mop your brow, you might want to wear proper cycling shoes with cleats so you can clip them onto the pedals. These are not essential but they are made for the job as they have stiff soles and good fixing points for the pedals. Trainers will suffice as most people who do spinning don't wear cycling shoes, they wear simple trainers. All the pedals have toe straps so all trainers fit in them easily. Cycling shorts are a luxury for me, some prefer gel seats because it can get a little uncomfortable when you first start to do spinning, but you do get used to it in time. Heart rate monitors are sometimes used. They are useful for seeing how hard you're working or to see if you're working at a certain intensity for you personally. I tend to think if you're breathless and sweating, that is a good sign as how hard you are working. So, if you go spinning and see some of the class chatting away effortlessly then think to yourself, they are probably doing it effortlessly!

Darren Salmon – *Manager of Longridge Civic Community Gym*
Qualified Gym Instructor, Personal Trainer, Kettle Bell Instructor, Circuit Instructor, Indoor Cycling Instructor, Fit2box Instructor

So that was spinning. Give it a go!

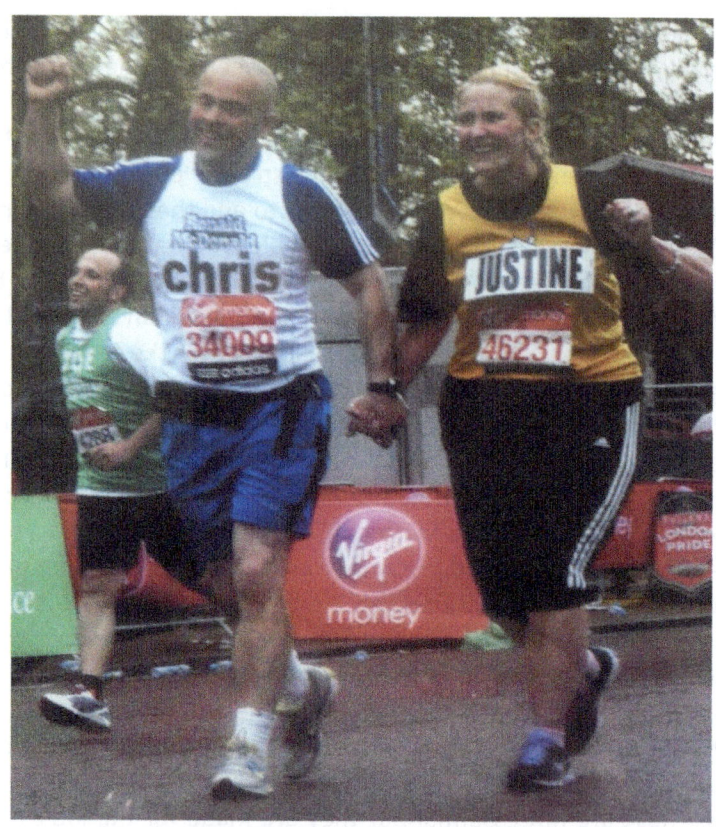

Running with Chris in the London Marathon 2012

RUNNING

I've just started running on the treadmill at the gym, doing interval training, and I love it! I try to do 30–60 minutes every other day.

Running outside is a totally different experience. I feel unsteady on my feet at times and a bit light headed. On the treadmill it's very comfortable and I don't feel breathless – until I stop running, that is.

After losing all the weight, my body doesn't weigh me down like before. I would never have been able to run if I was still carrying those extra 14 stones. I haven't run since my schooldays, when I really enjoyed long distance running, and I'm chuffed to be able to run once again. Every second I'm doing it, I'm smiling. That's because I am so happy at how far I've personally journeyed and I'm very proud of myself – there really isn't a better feeling in the whole world. Running on a treadmill is, in my opinion, easier than running on a road and better for your joints. The treadmill helps your legs and is low impact. You'll find that different muscles in your calves and the tops of your legs ache, but as they say: no pain no gain! I have to keep on top of my running. If I have a couple of weeks off, it takes a while to get back into it. I have a love/hate relationship with it. When I run outside I usually go with Chris, we seem to need each other to motivate ourselves. It's also nice to have someone to natter to if it's a long steady run. We've both run in the Great North Run and the London Marathon for our charity Ronald McDonald House, and will be repeating both. It's great to have such amazing goals to work to and I love the way I'm trying different things out, and sometimes the gym can become a little tedious if you don't inject variety into it.

As with most things: "Variety *is* the spice of life!"

Running indoor and outdoor by Mark Townsend

Indoor running:
Running on a treadmill indoors is a good way to train throughout the winter months, it also reduces the likelihood of injury because of the cushioning that the treadmill offers over road running. Although it delivers the same benefits, treadmill training is not quite the same as road running. If you fancy a go at treadmill training but have never used a treadmill before, then there are a few things you need to be aware of.

While you're running on a moving belt, your body is actually stationary relative to the air around you, which means there's no air flowing past your body. The downside to that is you will sweat more and feel hotter compared to outdoor running, so hydration is very important when running indoors and in warmer conditions. The plus side of treadmill running is that you tend to run a little faster for the same effort. Because treadmill running lacks the constantly changing scenery and environment as opposed to running outside, it can easily become boring. To try to overcome this you can perform a structured workout, i.e. hill programmes, interval speed sessions etc.

Outdoor running:
Running outdoors gets you into the fresh air, so it is likely to be better for your lungs than exercising indoors. Running outdoors is much harder on your joints than running on a cushioned treadmill and it is also harder to measure results, i.e. you may time yourself, but many factors can influence the time it takes you to complete your circuit, such as traffic or even walkers getting in your way. It's totally different to a treadmill, whereas measuring things is much easier to do, i.e. calories burned, distance covered, even

inclines and speed. To sum up the comparisons of a treadmill *v.* outdoor running, my own preference is that you cannot beat being outdoors with all the natural elements against you because it gives you that sense of freedom which running on a treadmill doesn't give. It is also very important to have the correct footwear and clothing to enable you to stay safe, whether you're running indoors or outdoors. One very important thing is, if you're thinking about running in the evening outdoors, is to be able to be seen. Be safe! Give them both a go and choose for yourself which one you prefer.
Mark Townsend – *Manager of Carter Leisure in Clitheroe*
Qualified Gym Instructor, Kettle Bell Instructor, Personal Trainer, Core Stability Trainer, Circuits Instructor, Spinning Instructor, Nutritional Adviser

SWIMMING

Next comes one of my very first loves – swimming! As you'll know from reading this book, I've done a lot of swimming in my time and love water. At my largest, it was difficult to visit public swimming baths because I had no confidence in myself and thought everyone was staring at me, which most people were. As a family, we've always enjoyed our holidays at Centre Parcs and one of the best things there are the swimming pools. I have to say they are the cleanest and nicest swimming facilities that we've ever come across, and that is one of the reasons we go back time after time.

Our kids love swimming too and have had private lessons from eighteen months old, it is such an important thing for children to learn, it is a life saver, after all!

Chris, on the other hand, hates water and anything to do with swimming. He had some lessons with the children's swimming instructor and improved his swimming and he had hoped this would help him to enjoy the water. Wrong! It didn't work; he still hates it and when we all go swimming we have to force him to come. I used to wonder how can someone go abroad for two weeks and not touch the swimming pool or the sea with their big toe, but after living with Chris for so long, I understand – he just doesn't like it!

When I joined the gym and was looking for different alternatives to the usual exercises one can do, I had an idea. I spoke with our children's swimming instructor, who owned the private pool where our children had their lessons, and negotiated pool hire for twice a week for an hour, for myself. It was great and it helped me out when I needed new ideas and alternatives to my exercise routine. I don't go now that I've started trying other exercises, and there is only so much time in a day. The other thing was that it was quite lonely, as I went by myself and late at night. I'm used to exercising to music and it was a killer for me not being able to listen to anything. Even when I'm walking Nell by myself, I've always got music on my headset. But swimming is a very healthy option and a good all over workout. However, if like Chris, you hate it, find something else instead that you really love to do.

ROWING

For me, this is my new "thing"! I love it at the moment and can't get enough of it. I can feel it really working my tummy muscles and making a difference to the appearance of my stomach. I've also got very competitive about it and put my times on the wall chart in the gym alongside other rowers. I aim to do 20 minutes rowing incorporated into other gym work, and try to go every weekday, leaving the weekends free, but I'm not obsessed with the gym and sometimes do give it a miss. How long I am there for depends on classes. Spinning classes, for example, are 45 minutes long, so I get there a little time before and do some rowing, then the spinning class, then home. I find it easier to do something before a class than after one, as I'm too tired afterwards.

I know I am very lucky because when I started on my journey into a healthier life, our oldest daughter Millie had reached an age where I was able to leave her in charge of Alex and Christopher, so that has been a real help because it's not that easy at times to find a sitter or someone who is able to take care of your children at short notice. Millie has helped me out in ways she'll just never understand.

KETTLE BELLS

This is a new fitness class that's just begun at our gym and is becoming popular. It started on a Thursday night after spinning with just a few of us behind to do it, but now there's lots more staying on for the class which lasts for half an hour. That half an hour is the quickest of the week for me, it just flies by. It consists of lots of reaches and stretches that incorporate your kettle bell weight. It really does strengthen and tone you up. It's also a good laugh too, which always helps the time fly.

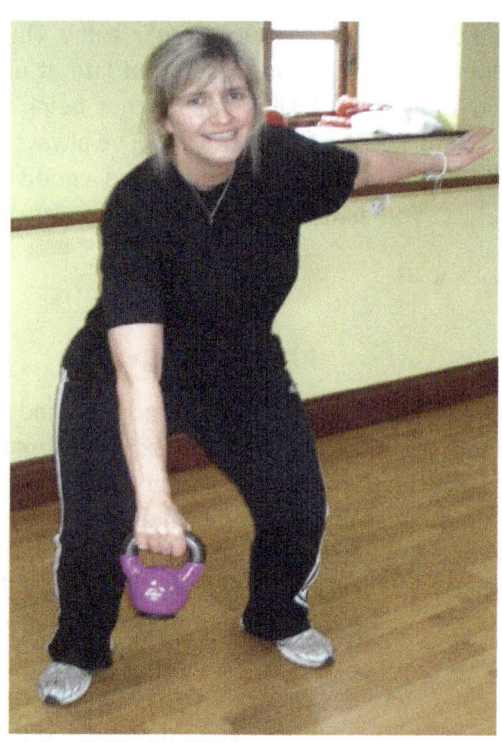

Kettle Bells by Darren Salmon

Kettle bells have been thrown about the fitness industry for a good few years now. Their origins go back to about 1704 when Russian soldiers used them to keep fit.

A kettle bell is basically a cannon ball with a handle on it; it sounds simple and it is, simple and very effective. It wasn't until the early 1900s that they became popular in other countries, mainly in America after a fitness magazine wrote a favourable article about them. The American army even employed a Russian to train their armed forces on how to use them after they noticed that their Russian counterparts were fitter and stronger.

Kettle bell workouts are usually about 20–30 minutes long, short but intense as most people that do kettle bells want a quick but intense workout and time is a key factor in this. Investing time and effort into something like kettle bells can make a huge difference in your health and wellbeing. Kettle bell training sees functional strength gain, which helps make everyday activities much easier. Your core and stabilizing muscles are challenged in kettle bells more so than in machine based exercises. You can't fire a cannon from a canoe, you'd need a solid base, and this sort of training can provide this. It gives you a strong and balanced body but not as bulky as some weight training can do. This is why a lot of sports people and celebrities have taken up this training. A mobile strong body is always helpful to any sports person.

The exercises we use are quite dynamic, as the main aspect of the sessions revolves around kettle bell swings, clean, clean and press, upright row, all of which involve squats thus improving legs, bum and back – the areas that most people want to work on. With these multi-muscle exercises the calories burned can be quite astonishing. It is also a great cardio workout as well as a strengthening workout. The kettle bell themselves range from 4k upwards. New people to a class will start with a light weight and then be instructed on the correct lifting techniques, shape and form with all the basic exercises, then progress to heavier weights and more challenging exercises as their fitness confidence and experience grows. Just three sessions a week could change your shape and fitness in a very short time. So what are you waiting for? Check out your local gym for details of their kettle bell classes.

WEIGHT TRAINING

Have you always been skinny or always overweight? Maybe you just want to tone and firm your body up? Then weight training is the one for you. Weight training builds a muscular body not to mention the other health benefits. Weight training is a proven life changer, it simply adds to your life. More people are weight training today and reaching their muscle building and weight loss goals than ever before. Now it's your turn. Don't let any more life pass away without at least trying this form of exercise.

CIRCUIT TRAINING

I have to admit I did give this a go. ONCE! I lasted 10 minutes, then walked from the class as I just found that I thought I couldn't do any of it. I'm very self-conscious in group classes, so most of them just aren't for me, especially when I feel I can't do certain forms of exercise. But I know there is no need to be self-conscious. Everyone is concentrating on their own performance and is too focussed to watch what you're doing. This also helps to keep you going and not look like you're giving up!

Circuit training has developed considerably over the years and this class is a fast-paced form of exercise suitable for anyone. Circuits can range from Boxercise classes to Body Pump – the main aim being to quickly develop the muscular system. After a warm up the class consists of a series of sports-specified exercises performed for a certain length of time, monitored and encouraged by an instructor. For toning, shaping and cardiovascular endurance there is no better class than circuit training.

ABS AND TONE

This is essentially a quick blitz class for the abdominal and lower back area and is very good for someone who wants to target that part of the body alongside their existing workout routine. Core stability is the key to all round fitness and you can achieve stronger, firmer and toned abdominal muscles by attending just one half-hour class once a week. Abs classes also use exercise balls to help stop you straining your neck when you're performing these exercises and also to create a higher intensity whilst focussing on your lower abdominal muscles.

These are some of the mottos you'll find in and around our gym. They've been put there to inspire and motivate you, I love reading them!

Where you begin doesn't matter, your willingness to start is what counts!

The pride you gain is worth all the pain.

Sports do not build character, they reveal it.

I've always felt it was not up to anyone else to make me give my best.

Motivation is what gets you started; habit is what keeps you going!

Nobody said it would be easy but everyone said it was worth it!

Exercise is like food, you cannot get enough in one sitting; it needs continuous and regular top ups!

Today is your day! Your mountain is waiting, so get on your way!

Everyone is different and may not enjoy the things I do, so give them all a go and decide for yourself because in the long run, that's half the battle, doing something you want to do because you enjoy doing it, it makes exercise so much more fun. People get involved in exercise for a number of reasons, the main one being to improve their health and physical condition or maybe to achieve a sporting ambition. Other people get involved in exercise to relieve themselves of the stresses of daily life or to lose some weight and change their lifestyle. The main thing we all tend to forget is that it is an essential part of our lives. For the way we look to the way we feel. We can all feel and look good by injecting a little health and fitness into our daily routine. You know it makes sense!

I love exercise, well, these days I do, but I didn't always. At the start of this amazing journey I hated it, but I could see how it worked and the benefits that can be gained. Just 30 minutes a day can make such a difference to your health and your life.

Look at me, I'm living proof!

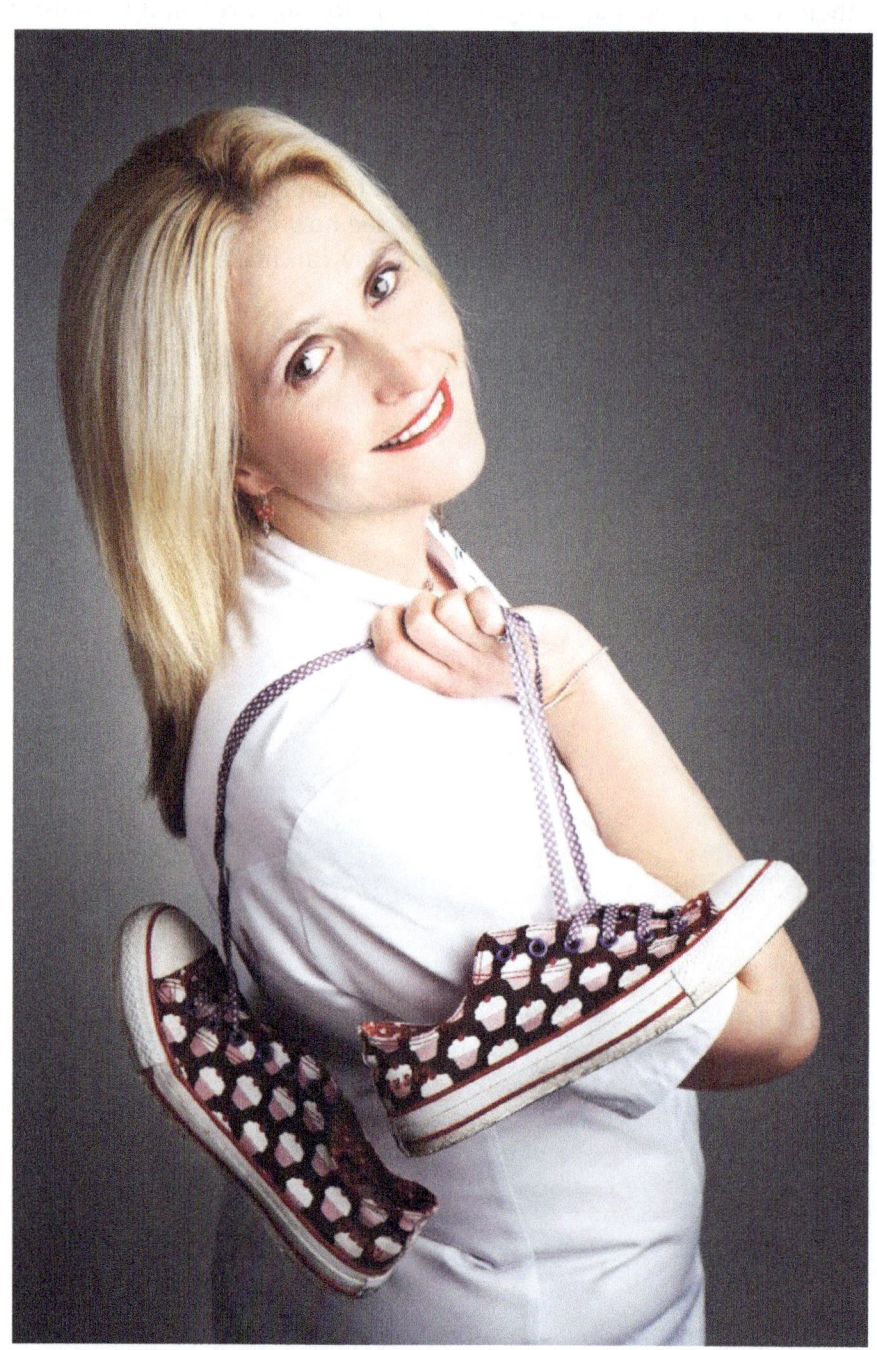

CHAPTER SIX

Who is Justine Forrest Today?

Who I am today and why losing weight has changed my life in every way possible.

Well, I don't really know where to start with this chapter because, apart from having the same personality as the Justine of old, I'm a completely different person but not only in the way I look.

Losing a massive amount of weight, in my opinion, is the biggest change that anyone can make. Everything has changed. The way I present myself, the way I walk, mix with people and the way I think. I now have so much more choice in everything I do and, of course, wear! I used to be judged straight away. People saw only a fat person and I found that I couldn't be taken seriously as it was so hard for some to get past my weight issue. First impressions seem to be very important in today's society and it can be bloody hard to cope with at times, even when it's a self-inflicted condition like obesity. People's first impressions and their perceptions of the person I am today are now *so* different. I'm not judged any more by my weight. When I meet someone for the first time, my weight is never discussed unless the conversation turns to dieting, and it usually does as everyone seems to be on a diet. Then people are astounded and some seem to go into a little shock and repeat "fourteen stone... You lost *fourteen stone*?"

I suppose one of the biggest changes is that I can now look forward to a future with my lovely family and set personal goals for myself. During the last four years, one of my goals was to start jogging, and now that I'm no longer lugging the extra pounds around with me, I can, at last, feel comfortable enough to run. Running had been an ambition of mine for over twenty years, and always a lifetime's ambition to run in a marathon, so you can imagine how ecstatic I am now to be doing just that. Chris and I ran in last year's Great North Run and the London Marathon. We're addicted to these marathons and half marathons, but nothing quite beats taking part in the London Marathon though, we loved it. What a difference a few years can make! Never in my wildest dreams did I ever think I would take part in either of these races. I remember always wanting to lose weight so that I could run in the London Marathon for my thirtieth birthday – well, that never happened. For years, I'd watched the London Marathon and the Great North Run and I secretly dreamt of competing. All those wonderful personal stories, the blood, sweat and tears that were shed and the heroes who went that extra mile, running such an amazing feat and all in the name of charity. Recently we were jogging up a steep road that several years before I struggled to walk along. When we reached the end, I ran hard all the way home with tears of joy, realising how far I had come in my own personal journey.

We've done all our runs for Ronald McDonald House, the charity close to our family's hearts. We've been lucky enough to experience the wonderful accommodation facilities that RMH offers alongside the Alder Hey Hospital in Liverpool, where Christopher had procedures and operations. Ronald McDonald House is a home from home for children and their families who have to stay in hospital for long periods of time. In having these wonderful facilities, it helps to keep all the family together and therefore helps the children's recovery. There are similar homes throughout the country – they make such a difference to the depressing and stressful situations the children and their families go through. I feel absolutely privileged that I can give something back to them as a way of saying a big THANK YOU for all they've done for us as a family.

I look back and think that not so very long ago, I struggled to walk for 10 minutes, never thinking that I would soon be running marathons. That's when I have to pinch myself. Chris and I plan to keep running marathons and in 2014, with Alex alongside, pushing our Millie around in her wheelchair, we will be raising money for Operation Smile, a cleft lip and palate charity.

These days I never think about dying and not making old age; those dark moments from my large days have disappeared. I'm in such good health and am so active and motivated, I truly believe anything and everything is possible, I'm living proof.

Let me tell you about my online business. Since being on the *Michael Winner's Dining Star*s TV programme, I'd been inundated with requests for my chocolate brownies and other home-made cakes. This gave me the confidence to set up *Brownies by Justine Forrest*, and I now make a whole range of hand-made cakes for mail order via my business website www.browniesbyjustineforrest.com, and for various retail outlets. It's very successful and I really enjoy having control over this income source. How my life has changed! I would never have considered this in my larger life. I'm delighted to say that every one of my customers approached me to supply them after hearing me on the radio or seeing me in different magazines and newspapers. I didn't have to go out touting for business.

It's amazing how all this has snowballed. I now have my own cake business, I run marathons for charity, write and give advice on healthy living at public speaking events, and regularly demonstrate at food events and festivals all over the country. Before, I would have never have had the courage to do this, and in my larger life it would have been impossible! Now, I stand on a stage and speak to a live audience, imagine! In the past, I couldn't even travel far on my own but now, I head off all over the country, up and down motorways as happy as can be. This is all down to the confidence I've gained from losing weight.

People often ask me how can I possibly bake and lose weight? WILLPOWER! That's how. It *is* possible to stay healthy and keep the weight off whilst baking wonderfully delicious cakes every day. If I can maintain my weight as I do and cook and bake all day with all these temptations staring at me, then I'm sure other people can too. For me, it's mind over matter and I'm used to it now. I don't think about food and cakes in the same way – I've retrained my brain and now I *eat to live* not *live to eat*.

My friends comment on the changes. They say I'm much more confident and that my personality has changed too. For example, I never carry a handbag. I used to always have a large bag gripped tightly across my body – I thought it hid my size! That only came to me the other day when I was out shopping and it was windy. My top was billowing out and I thought, God, I'd be pulling at my top by now and I'd feel mortified that everyone was watching me holding a silly bag to my tummy! The things you do… These days I don't even think about my clothes flapping around in the wind or my top not covering my stomach or my bottom any more.

Something else has happened in our household – my girls borrow my clothes! Just the other day I couldn't find one of my tops, then Millie walked in through the door wearing it! She'd pinched it from my bedroom that morning, but I couldn't be mad with her because inside me, I was secretly thrilled. Who'd ever have thought that my sixteen-year-old would want to wear some of my clothes – what a novelty!

I do so much more with my family now and am always eager to try new things and experience stuff I've never done before. I push myself to the limits and this is all down to my weight loss and having so much more confidence. Any challenge you want to throw my way, I'm having it! I'm obviously very sporty these days and love getting sweaty and feeling the adrenalin kick in and take over. I take a pride in everything I wear and love shopping for clothes – probably a little too much! I don't mind people looking at me either. When people used to look at the old Justine, I could tell they were thinking, "God, she's put some weight on or is she pregnant again?" I'd go anywhere on my own now, but the old Justine wouldn't have done. I hated gatherings and meeting people.

Valentine's Day recently was a whole new experience. I went shopping and bought ten beautiful matching underwear sets. I've gone down TEN sizes in my bras! I justified the expense by telling myself that they were a gift to Chris and amazingly, Chris fell for it and even agreed that they were the best presents he'd ever had from me. But really, deep down, it was a whole new thrilling experience for me as I can't ever remember buying any pretty underwear for myself. It used to be massive, black, belly warmer knickers that I'd had for years, in fact all of them had holes in and, I'm ashamed to say, were in a very sorry state. Undies were never a top priority and always the last thing I wanted to buy. There didn't seem much pleasure in buying and wearing a size 32 knick knacks or any size 46DD bra that would fit (that's if you could find them). I would stand there in the shop feeling a complete idiot and hating every moment. Now there's no stopping me. I just love buying new clothes and underwear. In fact, Chris and I feel like we are back in the honeymoon period. Not that Chris has ever been able to keep his hands off me, but now he's even worse! Friends of his ask him all the time: "What's it like to have a new wife?" Funny! But it's true – our sex life has never been better! When I was overweight it wasn't exactly an issue between us, mainly because we rarely made love. I just didn't enjoy it one little bit, it was so uncomfortable and painful for me. So you learn to do things differently or even not at all. But now we're like teenagers again and it's amazing, we're certainly making up for the last twenty years. Oh, and on the plus side... it's very good exercise. So – BONUS!

My Chris is amazing too and we support each other one hundred per cent. If there were ever a single thing in life that I can be sure about, then it would have to be Chris and myself. Nothing will ever split us up. We are soul mates and have never been as close; he is the best friend I've ever had and will ever have. No one will ever come between us; I know that for sure. We have been through far too much together and have come out the other end still loving and respecting each other, a rare commodity these days. We've been married for a long time, that's certainly some achievement.

I've experienced some pretty amazing things in the past few years and I'll always be grateful to Michael Winner for giving me the opportunity to experience some of these, and also to give me the chance to find myself and build on my courage, to take risks and show potential, as the great man himself put it. That show made me do everything for myself for the first time in my life, without hiding in anyone else's shadow. I had to think for myself and I even had to go through the pain of being isolated away from my precious family while I was away filming. I learnt so much. I always thought I was quite needy and couldn't do much by myself, but that was so untrue – it was just my weight holding me back, nothing else, just insecurities that came from me being morbidly obese. As I discovered, I *can* stand on my own two feet, I'm very independent and I'm driven when I want to be. I never thought that I was competitive, but in the right situation

– I am. I'm not useless, as I once thought, I love the way my new life rolls on and I just go with the flow. In the past, I had no confidence or self-esteem and would have hated change. Now, I love surprises and doing things at short notice and not having my life mapped out a year ahead. The old Justine lived through her family and her home, only because she didn't think much about herself. I still live for my family, nothing has changed in that respect, but they now stand independently on their own two feet for the first time in their lives, and because I just don't have the time to do everything, they have responsibilities and jobs. So, in turn, it's doing them good and equipping them for their future life. The old Justine vacuumed and cleaned the house daily, the new me doesn't really care! If I don't get time, it's not important any more. Time is so precious to me. When the kids look back on their childhood, do you think they'll say, "Oh, we had a lovely clean house when we were growing up", or will they remember all the exciting memories instead? Yes, I know, they'll remember all the fun stuff.

I find it satisfying that our children think about what they eat and how they exercise, without being obsessed about it. After being a part of my journey, they've gained incredible understanding on how to live a healthier life. I've never imposed my lifestyle changes on my family; they've made their own choices. I tell them that it's all about everything in moderation. You might think that they are too young to know any different but from my experience, children from a very young age can suffer weight issues and become obsessed about weight gain and calorie counting. I was brought up in an environment where calories were evil and weight gain totally unacceptable. My parents' understanding of weight issues was limited and as neither actually suffered from being overweight themselves, they didn't understand the issues I've had with food and how it affected my life.

I'm very passionate about teaching others and the next generation about the changes I've made to my lifestyle, as I believe it is such an important message in the world we live in and for generations to come. I want to inspire and help other people with their lifestyle issues. All my life I've had weight and eating problems, but now I've retrained the way I think about food and exercise and have helped to teach my children. I've experienced it from both sides and feel I know a lot of the issues we all go through every day, I want to share my invaluable knowledge. As parents, we have a responsibility to bring our children up in a healthy environment. Not only teaching them life's responsibilities and right from wrong, but also about different foods and healthy choices. We need to encourage our children to get outside and exercise, whether that's just a 20 minute walk or a visit to the swimming pool. All of these things should become a way of life, just like the air we breathe. I have three children and know that it's not easy at times, but we must make the effort. The way many live their lives now with all the computer games and takeaways on every street corner, we really need to teach our children about their healthy choices so that they, in turn, will teach the generations of children to come, otherwise obesity will get worse and be an even greater drain on our health service.

I wonder if my family would be as informed about healthy eating if I hadn't lost my weight? I guess I'll never know, but one thing is for sure – doing what I have done has shown them first hand the horrors of being massively overweight and how it gradually restricts and impacts on your life. It is totally self-inflicted. So take control! You *do* have the choice whether you overeat and don't exercise. *You* are in control! My family have been there and supported me through every stage, especially the grim and agonising skin removal surgeries. They've seen first hand what I've had to consequently put myself through because of over-eating for years. I hope that this will put them off living how I used to live my life and that they won't punish their bodies like I did. I wear the war wounds of pretty much a full body lift because of all the loose skin I was left with, my body is scarred all over simply because I ate too much. I'm happy with all my surgeries and grateful for the opportunity to have the sagging flesh removed, but it wasn't an easy option. For me it was a necessity, not for cosmetic reasons at all, especially the skin on my stomach. I had a very large apron, as the doctors described it, which got in the way and flapped around making it very uncomfortable to do anything. I wouldn't have been able to run before it was removed. Now it's gone, I don't have much feeling on my stomach, it's very scarred and I can't feel my belly button, but I'd much rather have it that way.

Another change has been in making new friends. I've been to so many new and different places and made lots of new friends, some quite famous too. Through my business and the food demonstrations I do, I roll with lots of chefs and other people that I would never have had an opportunity to meet in my larger life. At the gym I've made new friends close to home, so losing the weight has gained me lots of new friendships all round and I feel very fortunate.

Hair! Yes – I've been to a salon and had my hair styled. The last time I went to a hairdresser I was pregnant with Millie and I couldn't fit in the chair under the dryer. After that, I had to have someone come to my home to cut my hair, and that carried on for years. Now I love getting out and having my hair done inside a lovely salon instead of my kitchen! When I stopped going to the hairdresser and had someone come out to me, I used to say, "Well, it's so much handier them coming to me and cheaper." The real reason was, of course, that I felt humiliated and that everyone was staring at me in a salon. Now there's a whole new world out there for me. Can you see how losing the weight has changed my life completely? *Everything* is different, even the little things in life; everything is much easier and simpler. Every day is a joy and a pleasure and it's a wonderful thing to feel like that. Sometimes I am reduced to tears when a certain situation throws me back in time and reminds me of the way I used to be. I watched an advert recently showcasing a film about a very big woman. I was so embarrassed and upset because I was watching the old ME! The shock made me teary, just thinking about how far I've come and what I've achieved. It is, for me, pretty amazing! I know this may sound strange, but if you've ever experienced anything in life to that degree, you'll know exactly where I'm coming from.

On a lighter note, I really should get my life insurance policies reviewed! When we took them out many years ago, I remember being weighed while the insurance lady was filling out the forms. I was 25 stone! Crickey, that's why my premiums have always been sky high...

CHAPTER SEVEN

The Plan

This is my Plan – the routine I followed (and still do!) which led to my huge weight loss.

So now you are ready to start your new healthy lifestyle. The Plan I devised and followed is explained in this chapter.

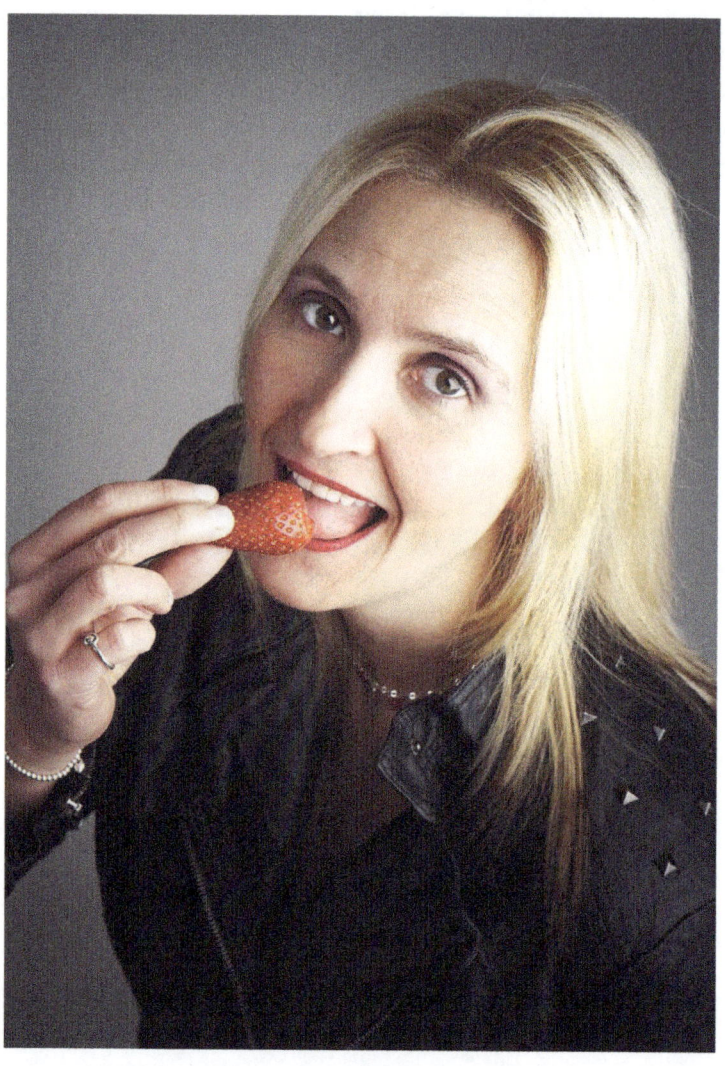

At the beginning, I followed my Plan for six whole weeks and didn't slip back into my old lifestyle once. After the six weeks, I slowly started to introduce some of my favourite foods into my everyday meals. Even today, I eat in the same way that I did when I first changed my lifestyle all those years ago, but unlike in the beginning, I now can make the choices for myself. Way back then, I had to consciously make the *right* choices if I wanted to live and not die a premature death because I was morbidly obese.

There are four main elements to the first six weeks of my Plan, my change of lifestyle (I'm not going to call it a diet; I hate the word "diet").

1. Eat healthy meals every day! Some will say, "What's so special about that?" Well, for most overweight people they all have one thing in common – skipping breakfast, the most important meal of the day.

2. Lunch with one of my healthy fresh smoothies! This was one of the biggest and most important changes I made, and even now I will sometimes have a smoothie instead of lunch when I'm trying to be super good.

3. Get moving! Plain and simple – I started walking and moving more. Anything that gets you a little hot and sweaty is exercise. When you're over 28 stone you're limited to what you can manage, so I chose walking as my exercise for the first year. It's free, you can do it anywhere, you don't need any special equipment and, most importantly, for me it wasn't dangerous for my colossal size.

4. Control your portions! I made sure that I ate before I got too hungry, ate smaller portions and only ate what was on my plate. It really helped me shift the pounds. Eating healthy meals with the family is a must in our home. I didn't want to set a bad example to my children by not enjoying mealtimes with them around our big kitchen table, or eating different things to them. It's all learning by example and I didn't want to bring them up with food issues too. Whenever I make a family size meal, such as lasagne, cottage pie, paella etc, I cover the leftovers straight away and put them in the fridge. That way, you're not cruising the dish for any more just because it's there and you can.

MY FIRST TWO WEEKS' HEALTHY LIFESTYLE PLAN

Everyone is different, so if there's a recipe you don't fancy or just don't like, then swop it for another. Nothing is set in stone and nothing is weighed or carefully measured. It's up to you how you stick to this Plan and it's all about managing these changes long term in your daily routine/lifestyle. You are the only one who can do this, so it's entirely up to you if you succeed or not. The closer you stick to my Plan the better it will work for you and the more weight you will lose. I've given you the tools, now it's up to you.

GET ORGANISED

I've written a daily list of foods you'll need, so check it at least the day before, to make sure you've got it in, or need it out of the freezer. I've also prepared a shopping list and a store cupboard list.

One of the big things I found extremely helpful with my Plan was making sure I knew what I was going to be eating a few days in advance. I made sure that I had bought in all the ingredients for my healthy meals, and once a week I would stock up my freezer with batches of my home-made meals, so I always had something ready.

Some of my recipes are family size, so you can either enjoy as a family together or once cooled down, freeze individual portions for the coming weeks. No one likes to eat the same meals every day, that's when the boredom can set in and you could find yourself straying back into all your bad habits.

With a little time and effort you can easily master this Plan. Even though I have always stated that you don't need to spend silly amounts of money on things for it, I would recommend you buy or borrow an electronic steamer. It's a great kitchen gadget. I try to steam most things, for example vegetables, chicken, fish and even some of my puddings. It makes food taste so much fresher and helps to hold in all their vitamins.

THE PLAN

Before you start the Plan do a little baking in advance. Yes, baking!

Baking: I want you to make one each of my delicious banana cake, bran cake, a batch of unfrosted carrot muffins and a batch of scones (you could buy medium size sultana scones if you don't have time to make all these cakes). Once you've baked the cakes, freeze them all into portions. That way, you'll only be eating the amount I've stated on each day and won't be tempted to have more. Cut the banana cake and bran cake into slices, roughly eight pieces to each cake and freeze each slice in separate freezer bags. They will also keep well in an airtight container for a week or two.

Daily Food List: Next, I've tried to make things a little easier for you by making a daily food list. You should check this the day before, so that you know you have all the ingredients for the next day's meals.

Store Cupboard List: I've compiled a store cupboard list for each of the two-week plans I've written for you (always remember, if you don't like a certain food or meal then simply swop it with another of my recipes; my two-week plan is only a guideline to show you how I got started and what worked for me). After the first two weeks you should be into a routine and you can start choosing from the rest of my recipes and making my Plan fit around YOU and what you enjoy eating.

Fresh Ingredients List: You'll also find a weekly fresh ingredients list. If possible, buy your fresh meat and fish the day before you need it. If that's not possible then I advise you to freeze your fresh meat and fish on the day of purchase. All the meal plan recipes state how many people they serve. Some will serve just two people; some will serve the whole family. It's up to you to either double the quantities of all the ingredients to make more, or cut the ingredients down to make less. Decide for each meal how many people you are catering for and adjust if necessary.

For the first six months of my weight loss journey I had one of my nutritious and filling fresh smoothies *every day* for my lunch. After six months, I started introducing what I would call "a proper lunch" into my meal plan. Remember, I had a colossal 14 stone in weight to lose and I was morbidly obese. I needed to stick to my smoothies for that length of time to give me the boost in weight loss. You're the only person who knows how much you want to lose, so you have to judge how long you think you need to have the meal replacement smoothies for. I would definitely recommend at least six weeks so your body and stomach can adjust to your new healthier food plan and smaller portions.

WEEK ONE

Your First Week's Store Cupboard List

1 box Bran Flakes
1 large box of All-Bran
1 box of Weetabix
1 bag porridge oats
1 bag sultanas
1 jar honey
1 jar raspberry jam
1 bag dried mixed fruit and nuts
1 bag dried apricots
1 bag mixed nuts
1 jar Worcestershire sauce
Tomato sauce
Mint sauce
1 jar mango chutney
Beef gravy granules
2 lamb stock cubes
3 fish/chicken or vegetable stock cubes
Salt/pepper
Low calorie fruit cordial (any flavour/flavours you fancy)
1 bag paella rice
1 bag couscous
1 jar smoked paprika
1 jar dried parsley
1 jar medium curry powder
1 jar ground cinnamon
1 jar medium chilli powder
1 jar cumin
1 jar lemon juice
1 large tin tomato soup
2 large tins reduced calorie baked beans
1 large tin kidney beans
1 large tin cannelloni beans
1 bottle white wine vinegar
1 bag brown sugar
Ingredients for banana cake, bran cake, carrot muffins, sultana scones – See Chapter Sixteen.

First Week's Fresh Ingredients List

Check out my smoothie recipes in Chapter Fifteen and pick one for your lunch each day. Choose the night before so you can make sure you have all the right ingredients ready to make one the next day.

4 apples
2 oranges
2 bananas
5 onions
2 whole heads of garlic
1 red onion
1 red pepper
1 green cabbage
5 low fat fruit yogurts of your choice
1 medium tub fromage frais
1 bag seedless green grapes
1 tub fresh tomatoes/cherry tomatoes
1 whole cucumber
1 lettuce or bag of mixed lettuce leaves
1 box mushrooms
1 bag white potatoes (ones perfect for mashing)
Skimmed milk (enough for breakfasts and hot drinks throughout the day)
1 small block of cheddar cheese
500g lean minced lamb
500g lean minced beef
3 carrots or 2 handfuls of frozen peas
1 packet of scones (if you're not making your own)
1 large bottle fresh orange juice
4 chicken breast fillets (split into 2x2 for 2 different recipes)
1 mixed packet of fresh fish bits, i.e. salmon, smoked haddock and cod. You can alternatively buy approximately 300g of fresh fish off cuts from your fishmonger or from your local supermarket, inexpensive bits will do.
1 bag fresh or frozen raw king prawns
2 salmon fillets
Vegetables: Choose lots of extra vegetables to have steamed most nights with your tea, e.g. sweetcorn (fresh/frozen), garden peas (fresh/frozen), swede, carrots, broccoli, cabbage, asparagus, mangetout. You can eat whatever vegetables you fancy and eat as much and as many as you can to "bulk" your plate out. No extra potatoes though!

DAY 1

Ingredients list for today's meal plan. This should be checked the night before so you can make sure you have all the necessary ingredients for all your meals throughout the day.

Ingredients list for the day

Bran Flakes
Skimmed milk
Sultanas
1 apple
1 low fat yogurt
1 orange
Mixed nuts
Sugar free fruit cordial/water to drink throughout the day, at least 8 glasses
500g lean minced lamb
3 carrots or 2 handfuls of fresh or frozen garden peas
Beef gravy granules
Mint sauce
Worcestershire sauce
3 cloves garlic
1 onion
6 mushrooms
Margarine
Cheddar cheese
2/3 bag of white potatoes for mashing
Extra vegetables for steaming, e.g. carrots, swede, sweetcorn, garden peas, broccoli, asparagus, mangetout
Salt/pepper
Smoothie: Fresh ingredients for your lunchtime smoothie, check out my recipes in Chapter Fifteen.

Menu for the day

Breakfast: 1 small bowl of Bran Flakes and warm or cold skimmed milk plus a dessertspoon of sultanas.
Midmorning Snack: 1 apple, 1 pot low fat yogurt.
Lunch: Choose from one of my fresh smoothie recipes from Chapter Fifteen.
Afternoon Snack: Handful of mixed nuts and 1 orange.
Tea: 2 serving spoons of my shepherd's pie, for recipe see Chapter Twelve. Lots of steamed vegetables, e.g. carrots, garden peas, broccoli, asparagus, mangetout, sweetcorn.

Exercise: For the first week I went for a brisk walk for 10–20 minutes every day after my breakfast; you can fit that into your daily routine anywhere and you MUST do it!

Drinks: I also drank coffee with skimmed milk, no sugar and unlimited water or low calorie cordial.

Nibbles: If you do get hungry really try to stay focussed and remember "no pain, no gain". Otherwise peel yourself a raw carrot to munch on.

DAY 2

Ingredient list for the day

1 scone (either home-made or shop bought)
1 dessertspoon raspberry jam
1 glass fresh orange juice
1 apple
1 banana
Sultanas
No sugar fruit cordial
One of my already baked, unfrosted carrot muffins
1 packet of mixed fresh fish bits, e.g. smoked haddock, salmon and cod
1 packet raw king/tiger prawns
300g paella rice
Smoked paprika
3 chicken/vegetable or fish stock cubes
Handful fresh or frozen garden peas
1 onion
3 cloves garlic
2 chicken breast fillets
Extra steamed vegetables, e.g. mangetout, sweetcorn, broccoli, carrots, asparagus, garden peas, swede
No sugar fruit cordial/water to drink – at least 8 glasses a day
Salt/pepper

Smoothie: Fresh ingredients for your lunchtime smoothie, recipes in Chapter Fifteen.

Menu for the day

Breakfast: 1 home-made or shop bought scone with 1 dessertspoon of raspberry jam, 1 apple, 1 glass of fresh orange juice.
Midmorning Snack: 1 banana, a handful of sultanas.
Lunch: Smoothie.
Afternoon Snack: 1 unfrosted carrot muffin.

Tea: 2 serving spoons of my paella, for recipe see Chapter Twelve. Steamed vegetables, e.g. sweetcorn, garden peas, mangetout, broccoli, cabbage.
Exercise: 10–20 minutes daily
Drinks: Lots of fluids! Flush you system!

DAY 3

Ingredient list for the day

Bran Flakes
All-Bran
Skimmed milk
Seedless green grapes
1 glass fresh orange juice
Ingredients for one of my lunchtime smoothie recipes (Chapter Fifteen)
Banana cake
1 apple
1 low fat fruit yogurt
2 chicken breast fillets
Sultanas
Seedless green grapes
Dried parsley
Mango chutney
Medium curry powder
Lemon juice
Low fat fromage frais
Salad ingredients: e.g. lettuce, tomatoes, red onion, cucumber, red or green pepper, sweetcorn
No sugar fruit cordial/water to drink, at least 8 glasses
Salt/pepper
Smoothie: Fresh ingredients for your lunchtime smoothie, check out my recipes in Chapter Fifteen.

Menu for the day

Breakfast: 1 small bowl of Bran Flakes with 1 dessertspoon of All-Bran and warm skimmed milk poured on top. A handful of seedless grapes, 1 glass of fresh orange juice.
Midmorning Snack: 1 slice of my banana cake (unbuttered).
Lunch: Fresh smoothie.
Afternoon Snack: 1 apple and 1 low fat yogurt.
Tea: My Coronation Chicken Salad, see Chapter Twelve.
Exercise: 10–20 minutes brisk walk.
Drinks: Unlimited fluids (sugar free).

DAY 4

Ingredient list for the day

Porridge oats
Sultanas
Skimmed milk
Honey
One orange
Mixed nuts
Banana cake
100g/4oz chipolata sausages
350g/12oz lambs liver
1 onion
1 large tin of tomato soup
1 large tin reduced calorie baked beans
Worcestershire sauce
White wine vinegar
Dijon mustard
Extra steamed vegetables, e.g. swede, broccoli, sweetcorn, garden peas, mangetout, cabbage, carrots
No sugar fruit cordial
Salt/pepper
Smoothie: Fresh ingredients for your lunchtime smoothie, see recipes in Chapter Fifteen.

Menu for the day

Breakfast: 1 big bowl of porridge made up by equal amounts of water and skimmed milk, a handful of sultanas and 1 dessertspoon of honey.
Midmorning Snack: 1 orange, 1 handful of mixed nuts.
Lunch: Fresh smoothie.
Afternoon Snack: 1 slice of my banana cake (unbuttered), recipe in Chapter Sixteen.
Tea: Liver, sausage and bean hotpot, for recipe see Chapter Twelve, served with steamed vegetables.
Exercise: 10–20 minutes brisk walk.
Drinks: Unlimited fluids (sugar free) at least 8 glasses. Try to drink as much water as possible.

DAY 5

Ingredient list for the day

2 Weetabix
Skimmed milk
Dried mixed fruit and nuts
1 low fat fruit yogurt
1 banana
Bran cake
2 salmon fillets
Ground cinnamon
Brown sugar
1 green cabbage
Extra steamed vegetables, e.g. carrots, sweetcorn, garden peas, broccoli, asparagus, mangetout
No sugar fruit cordial/water
Salt/pepper
Smoothie: Fresh ingredients for your lunchtime smoothie, see my recipes in Chapter Fifteen.

Menu for the Day

Breakfast: 2 Weetabix with warm skimmed milk and 1 small sliced banana on top.
Midmorning Snack: 1 handful of mixed fruit and nuts, 1 low fat fruit yogurt.
Lunch: Choose from one of my fresh smoothie recipes in Chapter Fifteen.
Afternoon Snack: 1 slice of my bran cake (unbuttered), see recipe in Chapter Sixteen.
Tea: Spiced sugar roasted salmon on a bed of cabbage, for recipe see Chapter Twelve, served with extra steamed vegetables, e.g. carrots, broccoli, mangetout, sweetcorn, steamed red peppers.
Exercise: 10–20 minutes brisk walk.
Drinks: Unlimited fluids (sugar free), at least 8 glasses. Try to drink as much water as possible.

DAY 6

Ingredients for the day

Porridge oats
Skimmed milk
Sultanas
Honey
1 glass fresh orange juice
1 of my unfrosted carrot muffins
Dried mixed fruit and nuts
1 low fat fruit yogurt
1 large tin kidney beans
1 large tin reduced calorie baked beans
1 large tin cannellini beans
500g/16oz lean minced beef
Chilli powder
Tomato sauce
Beef gravy granules
Worcestershire sauce
Garlic gloves
1 onion
6 mushrooms
6 large carrots
Unlimited no sugar fruit cordial and water
Salt/pepper
Smoothie: Fresh ingredients for your lunchtime smoothie, recipes in Chapter Fifteen.

Menu for the day

Breakfast: 1 bowl of porridge made up with equal quantities of water and skimmed milk, topped with a handful of sultanas and 1 dessertspoon of honey, 1 glass of fresh orange juice.
Midmorning Snack: Unfrosted carrot muffin, for recipe see Chapter Sixteen.
Lunch: Smoothie of your choice, see Chapter Fifteen.
Afternoon Snack: Handful of dried mixed fruit and nuts, 1 low fat fruit yogurt.
Tea: My recipe for a healthy three bean chilli con carne, see Chapter Twelve, served on a bed of steamed carrots.
Exercise: 10–20 minutes brisk walk.
Drinks: Unlimited fluids (sugar free), at least 8 glasses. Try to drink as much water as possible.

DAY 7

Ingredients for the day

1 scone (home-made or shop bought)
1 dessertspoon raspberry jam
1 glass fresh orange juice
1 apple
1 low calorie fruit yogurt
Sultanas
Banana cake
225g/8oz lean lamb steak
1 onion
3 cloves garlic
50g/2oz dried apricots
Cumin
2 lamb stock cubes
100g/4oz dried couscous
1 tablespoon fresh mint
A selection of steamed vegetables, e.g. carrots, broccoli, mangetout, asparagus, garden peas, sweetcorn
Unlimited no sugar fruit cordial/water
Salt/pepper
Smoothie: Fresh ingredients for your lunchtime smoothie, recipes in Chapter Fifteen.

Menu for the day

Breakfast: Home-made or shop bought fruit scone, topped with 1 dessertspoon of raspberry jam, 1 glass of fresh orange juice and 1 apple.
Midmorning Snack: 1 low fat yogurt and 1 handful of sultanas.
Lunch: Fresh smoothie.
Afternoon Snack: 1 slice of my banana cake (unbuttered), recipe in Chapter Sixteen.
Tea: Spiced lamb with couscous, recipe in Chapter Twelve, served with plenty of extra steamed vegetables, e.g. carrots, broccoli, asparagus, sweetcorn, mangetout, cabbage.
Exercise: Today, we're going to step up your exercise to at least 30 minutes daily for 6–7 days a week. If you want to exercise for longer, do so. This is how I planned my exercise. More is a bonus, less is a travesty!
Drinks: Unlimited fluids (sugar free), at least 8 glasses. Try to drink as much water as possible. This will not only keep you hydrated but will also help you feel fuller for longer. Get into the habit!

WEEK TWO

Your Second Week's Store Cupboard List

You'll probably find you have some of these ingredients left over from Week One. Just check if you have enough left to use in Week Two, if not replenish before you start.

All-Bran
Bran Flakes
Porridge oats
Weetabix
Honey
Sultanas
Mixed fried fruit and nuts
3 beef stock cubes
2 vegetable stock cubes
8oz dried brown rice
Raspberry jam
Brown sugar
Granulated sugar
Worcestershire sauce
Dark soya sauce
Tomato sauce
Cornflour
White wine vinegar
Lemon juice
Low fat mayonnaise
Whole grain mustard
Sweet chilli sauce
2 large tins chickpeas
3 large tins chopped tomatoes
1 tin of tuna in brine
1 small tin sweetcorn
1 large tin water chestnuts
1 large tin butterbeans
Turmeric
Dried ground coriander
Medium chilli powder
No sugar fruit cordial
Salt/pepper
Ingredients for banana cake, bran cake, carrot muffins, sultana scones – see Chapter Sixteen.

Cakes: Check that you have enough cakes left to see you through another week. If you don't, bake some more in advance and stock up your cake tins. All these cake recipes are old family favourites of ours, so even though you're restricting yourself to only eating one slice at a time, who knows what the rest of the family are sneaking away behind your back. I consider these amongst the healthiest cakes to bake that are still full of flavour and very tasty, but sort-of good for you at the same time!

Second Week's Fresh Ingredients List

100g button mushrooms
300g/12oz mushrooms
175g/6oz courgettes
Plus 2 extra courgettes
2 large beef tomatoes
2 large white potatoes
4 sticks of celery
6 spring onions
8 apples
3 bananas
2 plums
1 red cabbage
2 bulbs garlic
1 pear
1 green pepper
1 red pepper
Seedless green grapes
1 whole fresh ginger root
Fresh basil
1 bag mixed stir fry vegetables
1 bag bean sprouts
1 bag fresh noodles – you'll find these with the fresh stir fry vegetables in the supermarket veg aisle
450g/1lb lean pork fillets
2 lean frying steaks
500g/1lb 4oz lean steak mince
Cooked (2 in a pack) sweet chilli salmon fillets – you'll find these in the fish section of the supermarket. If you can't find them, then plain cooked salmon fillets will do.
2 eggs
Medium sized block of edam cheese

300g/10½oz low fat Greek yogurt
175g/6oz low fat fromage frais
3 low fat fruit yogurt pots
1 low fat natural yogurt pot
1 bag medium frozen prawns
Fresh orange juice
Skimmed milk
No sugar fruit cordial of your choice
Smoothies: Fresh ingredients for your lunchtime smoothies, see recipes in Chapter Fifteen.
Home-made or shop bought fruit scones.
Extra vegetables for steaming, e.g. sweetcorn, mangetout, carrots, broccoli, asparagus, swede.
A selection of salad vegetables to eat with your cold meals, e.g. little gem lettuce or a bag of mixed salad leaves, tomatoes, cucumber, red onions, green, red or yellow peppers, sweetcorn.

DAY 1

Ingredients for the day

Porridge oats
Skimmed milk
Honey
Sultanas
1 apple
Dried mixed fruit and nuts
Smoothie ingredients for you lunch
Bran cake
2 tins chickpeas
1 onion
1 tin chopped tomatoes
1 clove garlic
2 vegetable stock cubes
½ teaspoon ground coriander
1 teaspoon medium chilli powder
225g/8oz dried brown rice
225g/8oz sliced mushrooms
No sugar fruit cordial/water
Lots of steamed vegetable, e.g. swede, carrots, sweetcorn, mangetout, broccoli, asparagus
Salt/pepper

Smoothie: Fresh ingredients for your lunchtime smoothie, check out my recipes in Chapter Fifteen.

Menu for the day

Breakfast: 1 big bowl of porridge made up with equal amounts of skimmed milk and water, topped with 1 dessertspoon of honey and a handful of sultanas.
Midmorning Snack: 1 apple and a handful of dried fruit and nuts.
Lunch: Smoothie.
Afternoon Snack: A slice of my bran cake (unbuttered), for recipe see Chapter Sixteen.
Tea: Spicy chickpea casserole served with a portion of brown rice, see my recipe in Chapter Twelve.
Exercise: At least 30 minutes of your chosen exercise.
Drinks: Unlimited fluids (sugar free), at least 8 glasses. Try to drink as much water as possible and ensure you're still hydrating yourself throughout the day.

DAY 2

Ingredients of the day

Bran Flakes
All-Bran
Skimmed milk
2 plums
1 banana
1 low fat natural yogurt
Honey
Seedless green grapes
2 large beef tomatoes
1 tin of tuna in brine
½ onion
50g/2oz edam cheese
Extra vegetables for steaming, e.g. sweetcorn, carrots, broccoli, asparagus, mangetout, cauliflower
No sugar fruit cordial
Salt/pepper
Smoothie: Fresh ingredients for your lunchtime smoothie, check out recipes in Chapter Fifteen.

Menu for the day

Breakfast: 1 bowl of Bran Flakes topped off with 1 dessertspoon of All-Bran and skimmed milk.
Midmorning Snack: 2 plums and 1 banana.
Lunch: Fresh smoothie.
Afternoon Snack: 1 natural yogurt topped off with a handful of halved grapes and 1 teaspoon of honey.
Tea: Tuna stuffed beef tomatoes, for recipe see Chapter Twelve, served with either a large side salad or lots of extra steamed vegetables.
Exercise: At least 30 minutes exercise to get that body of yours moving and to burn those calories and get you fit.
Drinks: Unlimited water or low calorie cordial throughout the day.

DAY 3

Ingredients for the day

Sultana scone (shop bought or home-made)
1 dessertspoon raspberry jam
1 glass fresh orange juice
1 banana
1 unfrosted carrot muffin (see Chapter Sixteen for recipe)
Seedless green grapes
Salad vegetables, e.g. little gem lettuce, mixed salad leaves, sweetcorn, tomatoes, cucumber, red onions, red or green pepper, cherry tomatoes
2 cloves garlic
1 onion
2 courgettes
2 large white potatoes
500g/1lb 4oz lean steak mince
1 beef stock cube
Worcestershire sauce
1 large tin chopped tomatoes
300g/10½oz low fat Greek yogurt
30g/2oz edam cheese
No sugar fruit cordial
Salt/pepper
Smoothie: Fresh ingredients for your lunchtime smoothie, recipes in Chapter Fifteen.

Menu for the day

Breakfast: 1 home-made or shop bought scone topped off with 1 dessertspoon of raspberry jam, 1 glass of fresh orange juice and 1 banana.
Midmorning Snack: 1 of my unfrosted carrot muffins, recipe in Chapter Sixteen.
Lunch: Fresh smoothie.
Afternoon Snack: Handful of seedless grapes and 1 apple
Tea: 2 serving spoons of my home-made moussaka, for recipe see Chapter Twelve, served with a large side salad.
Exercise: Don't forget your 30 minutes of exercise. If you can do a little more, then do.
Drinks: Lots and lots of fluids in the form of water or low calorie cordial throughout the day.

DAY 4

Ingredients for the day

2 Weetabix
Skimmed milk
Sultanas
1 glass fresh orange juice
Banana cake – for recipe see Chapter Sixteen
1 low fat fruit yogurt
3 apples
Lemon juice
4 sticks celery
6 spring onions
1 large tin butterbeans
175/6oz low fat fromage frais
White wine vinegar
½ teaspoon turmeric
Granulated sugar
No sugar fruit cordial
Salt/pepper
Smoothie: Fresh ingredients for your lunchtime smoothie, see my recipes in Chapter Fifteen.

Menu for the day

Breakfast: 2 Weetabix with warmed skimmed milk and a handful of sultanas on top, 1 glass of fresh orange juice and 1 apple.
Midmorning Snack: 1 slice of banana cake (unbuttered).
Lunch: Fresh smoothies.
Afternoon Snack: 1 low fat fruit yogurt, 1 apple.
Tea: Waldorf salad, for recipe see Chapter Twelve.
Exercise: 30 minutes exercise at least.
Drinks: Unlimited water or low calorie cordial.

Tip: I try to carry a water bottle around with me everywhere, that way I can always have a drink.

Tip: If you need a sweet "hit" try a low calorie hot chocolate drink.

DAY 5

Ingredients for the day

Porridge
Skimmed milk
Honey
1 glass fresh orange juice
1 apple
1 low fat fruit yogurt
Banana cake (see recipe in Chapter Sixteen)
Extra steamed vegetables, e.g. broccoli, cauliflower, asparagus, carrots, sweetcorn, swede, mangetout
3 cloves garlic
100g/4oz button mushrooms
1 onion
450g/1lb lean pork fillets
175g/6oz courgettes
1 green pepper
1 large tin chopped tomatoes
2 beef stock cubes
1 tablespoon chopped basil
No sugar unlimited fruit cordial to drink throughout the day
Salt/pepper
Smoothie: Fresh ingredients for your lunchtime smoothie, see recipes in Chapter Fifteen.

Menu for the day

Breakfast: 1 bowl of porridge made up with equal amounts of skimmed milk and water, topped with 1 dessertspoon of honey, 1 glass of fresh orange juice.
Midmorning Snack: 1 low fat fruit yogurt and 1 apple.
Lunch: Fresh smoothie.
Afternoon Snack: 1 slice of banana cake (unbuttered).
Tea: Pork ragout, for recipe see Chapter Sixteen, plus lots of extra steamed vegetables, e.g. carrots, broccoli, cabbage, mangetout, garden peas, sweetcorn, cabbage.
Exercise: Don't forget to do at least 30 minutes exercise, 6–7 days a week.
Drinks: Keep drinking plenty of fluids in the form of water or low calorie cordials.
Tip: Try to moderate your alcohol intake – a glass of wine is fine but alcohol weakens your willpower!

DAY 6

Ingredients for the day

2 Weetabix
Skimmed milk
1 banana
1 glass of fresh orange juice
Mixed dried fruit and nuts
1 apple
1 unfrosted carrot muffin, for recipe see Chapter Sixteen
Fresh root ginger
Brown sugar
Dark soya sauce
2 lean frying steaks
1 bag mixed stir fry vegetables
1 bag of fresh noodles
½ bag bean sprouts
1 onion
3 cloves garlic
White wine vinegar
Tomato sauce
Cornflour
6 mushrooms
1 tin of water chestnuts

Unlimited no sugar fruit cordial
Salt/pepper
Smoothie: Fresh ingredients for your lunchtime smoothie, check out my recipes in Chapter Fifteen.

Menu for the day

Breakfast: 2 Weetabix with skimmed milk and topped off with 1 small sliced banana. 1 glass of fresh orange juice.
Midmorning Snack: 1 handful of mixed dried fruit and nuts, 1 apple.
Lunch: Fresh smoothie.
Afternoon Snack: 1 unfrosted carrot muffin.
Tea: Healthy stir fry, for recipe see Chapter Twelve.
Exercise: At least 30 minutes exercise. You can choose when it's your rest day.
Drinks: Lots and lots of lovely hydrating water or low calorie cordial throughout the day.

DAY 7

Ingredients for the day

Bran Flakes
All-Bran
Skimmed milk
1 apple
1 glass of fresh orange juice
1 pear
1 low fat fruit yogurt
1 of my unfrosted carrot muffins, see recipe Chapter Sixteen
Large mixed salad: mixed lettuce leaves, tomatoes, cherry tomatoes, red onion, red or green pepper, sweetcorn, cucumber
Sweet chilli salmon fillet
1 bag of frozen medium prawns
½ red cabbage
1 onion
3 carrots
3 tablespoons low fat mayonnaise
1½ teaspoons chilli powder
2 tablespoons whole grain mustard
2 tablespoons sweet chilli sauce
Unlimited no sugar fruit cordial/water

Salt/pepper
Smoothie: Fresh ingredients for your lunchtime smoothie, Chapter Fifteen.

Menu for the day

Breakfast: 1 bowl of Bran Flakes with a dessertspoon of All-Bran on top, finished off with warm skimmed milk, 1 apple and 1 glass of fresh orange juice.
Midmorning Snack: 1 low fat fruit yogurt and 1 pear.
Lunch: Fresh smoothie.
Afternoon Snack: 1 unfrosted carrot muffin and a handful of seedless grapes.
Tea: Salmon and prawn salad, see Chapter Twelve, with lashings of my low fat spicy slaw, see Chapter Twelve.
Exercise: Don't forget your 30 minutes of daily exercise. This is extremely important for keeping to a healthy lifestyle change and losing weight.
Drinks: Unlimited water or low calorie cordial all day.

Tip: Smoothie – if you are going out for the day or taking this to work for lunch, store in a container placed in a cooler bag, and choose one of the smoothies that keeps well from the list mentioned in Chapter Fifteen.

Coffee: I have one really bad habit – I drink way too much coffee and couldn't live without the brown stuff. I do try to limit it and drink it with skimmed milk and no sugar. All those little changes helped. If you can make the change to decaffeinated coffee and tea, it can help to keep your cholesterol in check.

I hope my sample meal plans help and that you read through my recipes and start to choose meals that you fancy. Don't forget you can substitute any meals for others listed in the later chapters. Don't be scared to mix things up a little.

After cutting out pasta and bread *completely* for my first 6 weeks, I began to introduce them back into my diet. After 6 months, I also started to substitute my fresh healthy smoothies for other light, healthy lunches. Try the changes for the initial 6 weeks, to allow you to get used to them and fit them into your routine.

CHAPTER EIGHT

Top Tips and Handy Hints

Little things that will hopefully help you build up a healthy way of thinking for yourself and give you the tools to make the right choices in your life.

I am sure that you've heard of some of these tips before. I've used them all at some point and some of them I still swear by to this day.

Everyone is different, so what works for me won't necessarily work for you, but if you use some of the things I've listed below, mixed together with some common sense and willpower, I'm hoping that they'll also work for you. If I can do it – anyone can, it's all about how much you want to achieve it.

Believe in yourself and make the changes!

One of the first things people ask me is: *"How have I done it?"* Well, sadly, there's no secret or a magic wand, but I do have six top things that I changed in my lifestyle when I seriously started to want to lose weight and alter my life.

It's simple. I think people make much more of a deal than it needs to be.

Further down this list I will revisit all six of them in more detail but, first, this is my sample list for you to skim over.

Top Tip 1
Portion control is crucial! Don't eat large platefuls at every mealtime. Get into the habit of choosing smaller portions.

Top Tip 2
Exercise! The most important thing you can do is inject a little gentle exercise into your daily routine and lifestyle. That doesn't mean busting your butt at a gym with a personal trainer, it may be by going for a 20 minute brisk walk each day.

Top Tip 3
Smoothies! For the first couple of months I would recommend that you swop your lunch for one of my healthy smoothies, just as I did. You get a lot of your daily vitamins and nutrition from one of these babies. The big thing for me was that I found it easier to *drink* my lunch in a liquid form instead of eating a meal and then finding I couldn't stop nibbling for the rest of the afternoon.

Top Tip 4
Plan your meals! Always plan your meals at least a day in advance, that way you'll always have something to look forward to and know exactly what you're going to be eating and it will be ready just as soon as you need to eat.

Top Tip 5
Bin your scales! I know this sounds extreme but I would recommend that you only weigh yourself once a month. Take your weight and all over measurements at the beginning of your journey. Get someone to hide your bathroom scales or move them to somewhere you can't get to them. Scales mess with your mind BIG style! Weighing-in once a month is enough – trust me.

Top Tip 6
Eat breakfast! It has to be the oldest one in the book, but to me it's certainly the most important top tip. *Always* eat a healthy breakfast, never, *ever* leave the house without breakfast in your tummy. It sets you up for the day and will help you lose weight.

Now you've sampled my quick start top tips for weight loss and managing your weight, read on for my more detailed list, for you to pick through and follow.

1. Digest your food properly.
Don't rush any of your meals – take your time eating. If you still feel hungry after eating what you think is enough, wait half an hour. I can promise you that however hungry you were, within half an hour you'll feel much fuller; as your food starts to digest you'll no longer feel the need to eat anything else. Think about when you fly – the flight attendants bring around a meal for everyone and they look so small, but they actually fill you up because, in general, our eyes are much bigger than our bellies and we think we need massive portions of food when actually a smaller portion will suffice.

2. Plan your meals in advance.
Always try to do this; it saves time and stops you reaching for the nearest thing to eat because you've got too hungry to wait. I always found, especially in the beginning, that if I left it too late to eat, or tried not to eat for a long period of time, I got way too hungry and was in danger of eating anything and everything. If I planned meals, there was always something healthy ready for those hectic times. Knowing what I'm going to be eating a

couple of meals in advance has really helped me, and meal planning for several days in advance is still something I try to do. It stops you wasting food, and you know that you and your family will be getting something nutritious and healthy at meal times.

3. Food rule.
My food rule and it's entirely up to you if you choose to use it. I cut out some food groups from the start of my journey. These were potatoes, pasta, cheese and bread. For a treat, I would eat a little cheese in a lasagne etc. I'm a cheese freak, and if there's one food I could choose to take with me to a desert island it would have to be cheese. Cheese goes with everything and I couldn't totally live without it forever, but when I'm being really conscientious about what I eat, I try to give cheese a miss as it is high in calories and fat. The whole thing about healthy living is being aware of what you put into your mouth. At times it can seem complicated having to think about every little thing that you're eating, but it does get easier and becomes second nature in the end.

4. Tight jeans.
Another top tip that I use when I feel I've over indulged and need to get back on track, is to get into some tight fitting jeans to remind me how awful I feel in my clothes when they don't fit me as they should. It works every time.

5. Seasoning when cooking.
Healthy low fat food can be a little tasteless, so a top tip I use is to always season my food at the start of any cooking process to ensure I bring out as much of the flavour as possible. Previous to starting my plan, I never used to do this, as I thought you just didn't need it and that added salt was bad for you. I've done a complete U-turn. I now think that when you're cooking healthy, plain foods you need to enhance them as much as possible. Seasoning is a very effective way of doing this because salt brings all the flavours out.

6. Don't measure everything.
Don't calorie count or measure and weigh all your food. This is your way of life now; you're retraining yourself to know your own portion control and what's right and what's wrong for you. This has to be manageable and you have to be in control for this to work. There's no need to make it complicated in any way because for you to stick to this plan, it has to be simple to follow.

7. Hide your bathroom scales.
There is no doubt that you do need to keep a record, but how you do this is up to you. I recommend that you only weigh yourself once a month, or every couple of weeks at the most. Don't be a slave to the scales. Judge by how you feel in your clothes, how well in general you feel within yourself. I weighed once a month, it was always a nice surprise to see the pounds going down. I didn't want to be dictated to by my weighing scales because it had never worked for me in the past. I had years of feeling really, really bad if I hadn't lost any weight when I weighed myself, and feeling awful if I'd only lost a few miserable pounds. So I decided to go by the way I felt and looked in the mirror. I weighed myself initially, but mainly to shock myself into changing my lifestyle. I then got Chris to hide the scales in the loft. This was the only place in the house I'd never go to as I couldn't get up the loft ladder, so they were going to be very safe up there! I do have one regret though, and that was I didn't take any photographs or measure myself from the beginning. I strongly suggest you do this when you begin your journey. I'm now a strong advocate that it's how you look and feel in your clothes and not all about what the weighing scales say. I measured my weight loss in dress sizes, a size 32 when I started, and now I'm a size 12–14. Nor did I do it through weighing at slimming clubs. These clubs are obsessed with weighing you every week; I think it's awful and doesn't work for everyone. I have friends who have been going to some of these clubs for years and years and they're still the same weight as when they started. One of the main reasons I never went to a diet club was the whole weighing thing and having someone write it down – the thought sends me into a complete frenzy!

8. A thought I keep in my head.
Whenever I'm not very motivated, I think to myself *"nothing tastes better than feeling good in your clothes!"* How true that is, and that thought gets me back on track.

9. You've got to really want it!
Yes, you've got to really want it for yourself to succeed. No one else can do it for you. It's not been any easier or any harder for me, but I've achieved it because I've wanted it more than the person next to me who hasn't achieved it.

10. You're not on a diet!
Don't tell yourself or other people that you're on a diet, because you're not. You're changing your lifestyle and living a healthier one. Dieting sounds so

horrid, so I never use the word and don't like the way people talk about dieting. There is a real problem with obesity and other food related illnesses. I believe some of this is because of the way we tackle it as a society, how we label it as a "diet", and that we should all be on one if we're overweight. Obesity needs to be tackled by a healthy lifestyle change and should be approached as such. It needs to be promoted in that way to encourage people to change their lives, not to scare them into thinking they could never achieve it. Dieting sounds so short term and unmanageable, but a change of lifestyle is something that can be maintained and managed long term. It's all about healthy living, and I portray it that way because that's what my family and I are now doing. I would hate to talk about dieting in front of my children because I don't want them growing up with any issues concerning food such as I had when I was younger. Children don't understand it's not a diet, it's a change of lifestyle, and that's what it should be called – a lifestyle change. Choosing the right foods to eat and doing some kind of exercise shouldn't be a chore, it should just be a natural way of life.

11. Fat pictures.
As soon as I started losing some weight I started collecting fat pictures of myself. That was no mean feat as I was always the one taking the photographs, so I wouldn't be seen on any them. Every large person will identify with that one, I'm sure. I now have a large collection of shocking fat pictures of myself that I'm, strangely, actually very proud of. Most of them were taken by our best friends, Simon and Nik. Simon has documented my weight loss through photos he's taken of me over the years. I even have one of me as a dinner lady at my little boy's school. I make all the other dinner ladies look tiny. Not only was I very wide at that stage, I'm actually quite tall at 5 foot 11 inches. It's strange, because since losing the weight, people have often said that I seemed to have grown taller; that's because I'm not as wide any more, surely? The dinner lady photo must be my worst picture ever, but I've had it enlarged and laminated to remind me of how truly awful I looked. That for me is a top tip: pick a cupboard. I chose the one that we used to keep chocolate and biscuits in and I've stuck loads of these photos on it. What an incentive to never go back!

12. Don't set your goals too high.
Set manageable targets; if you set them too high you've more chance of failing. I never started out thinking I could lose 14 stone in 18 months. If I had, I doubt I would have done it because that sounded too much to tackle, and I couldn't, or didn't, want to accept I had that much weight to lose in

the first place. I started out by wanting to lose baby weight, which was roughly 5 stone. I set myself little targets, then thought about what I would buy myself as a reward for reaching those goals. They would be jewellery treats usually, or clothes – nothing foodie! Having dropped so many clothes sizes, at one stage it seems clothes were all I bought. It was lovely to buy a size or two smaller and hang it in my wardrobe to give me the extra incentive to carry on and get into it. Having something in mind was very exciting, and knowing I'd earned it by doing really well was even more precious for me on my downsizing journey.

13. Lunch replacement smoothies.
For about the first 6 months, to kick-start my healthy lifestyle I replaced my lunch most days with one of my healthy smoothies. I also found that if I was out for the day my smoothies were really handy to take with me and have while on the move. They really sustained me until teatime. My weight dropped off. I use my smoothies even now from time to time as a meal replacement when I don't feel like eating a big meal.

14. Not eating after 6:00 pm.
I did this from the start and still do it to this day. I don't ever get hungry at night any more, which is very strange because that's when I used to do most of my eating. Set a time, say, 6:00 pm. I try not to eat after 5:00 pm now. Most days, I have my main meal at lunchtime as this gives me all day to work it off. Do try really hard not to eat in the evening as it's the worst time of the day to digest your food and will lie heavy on your stomach while you're sleeping at night.

15. Swop some foods.
When you go out food shopping, replace all your white foods with brown. White rice for brown rice, white pasta for brown pasta, white bread for brown bread – every white food that has a brown alternative, replace it. It's a small change, but it makes it a much healthier one, and knowing that your family is also making the changes without even noticing, makes it even better.

16. Buy yourself the best foods you can afford.
This is a very good tip. When you're limiting your food and choosing the healthier option, I would suggest that you indulge in the best types of food you can afford. With all the savings on the quantities you now eat, you can afford to pay a little more. For example, I love sushi so I buy a lot of it for my lunches, and I wouldn't necessarily buy sushi for all the family because it's

quite expensive and not everyone in my family likes it. I also buy a lot of good quality prawns as they are low in calories and I love them, but again they are expensive, but when you're only buying for yourself for lunch, you can afford it. Go on, treat yourself! Spend a little extra on what takes your fancy.

17. Brushing your teeth.
I like this tip. Clean your teeth straight after eating. If I'm out I'll have a mint instead, which works just as well. Chewing gum is another one, but whatever you choose, make sure it's sugar free.

18. Cutting back.
For the first couple of months, I started off removing certain foods from my diet one at a time, over a long period of time. These little changes do make a difference and if you do it one thing at a time, it makes it far more manageable. I used to love cola, in fact I was addicted to it, as I'm not a big tea drinker and I also don't like the taste of alcohol. First, I replaced cola with a sugar free version and then eventually cut it out all together. I did the same with butter, sugar, crisps, pasta, bread and cheese, along with biscuits, cake and any other unhealthy snack. Do it slowly. You'll find that you really won't miss any of them.

19. Leftovers.
Never ever nibble on leftovers of any description. Leftovers are evil! I've tried but I can't resist. I'm fine if I deal with them straight away and throw them straight into the bin, but if I stumble for a moment and have a quick nibble, I succumb to the lot. Once I get that taste, I just can't resist. So I keep to my rule to completely ignore leftovers. That way, there's no temptation for me to finish off and eat any more calories.

20. Learn to accept who you are.
Accepting your body faults and imperfections is half the battle in trying to achieve a new healthier way of life. Work with what you have and not what you wished you had! Then any body changes, even the smallest ones, will help empower you and give you more confidence.

21. Labelling.
Don't assume that when you're out shopping everything that says "low fat" or "fat free" on the label is automatically going to be a lot better for you. Some supermarket labelling is very misleading, so read it very carefully and try to understand it. For a rough guide, I always look for the calorie content

in the products and what that gives you for the portion size. Also look for how much saturated fat a product has in it, you're looking for it to be low.

22. Drink lots of water at meal time.
Drinking lots of cold water along with your meal fills your stomach and makes you feel a whole lot fuller. Try to meet the target of at least 8 glasses a day. Water is also wonderful for your completion.

23. Try to choose lots of low GI foods.
Try to incorporate as many GI foods into your daily food intake as you can as they result in lowering your insulin levels, which makes fat easier to burn and less likely to be stored. Low GI foods are found in multigrain breads, rolled oats, muesli, apples, citrus fruits, sweet potatoes and sweetcorn.

24. Cut down on alcohol.
If you're trying to lose weight, cut down on your alcohol intake or, better still, give it a miss altogether. Alcohol has so many hidden calories and bloats you, it gives you a beer belly too. Cutting it out will not only help shift some weight but will also make you look and feel much better.

25. Don't go exercise crazy.
Doing too much exercise can be as bad for you as doing too little. I don't exercise every day but I do it more often than I miss not doing it. It's an 80/20 per cent thing. If you're good and focussed 80 per cent of the time then you can be naughty for the remaining 20 per cent. It's all about knowing when to stop! Exercising also keeps your metabolic rate up which, in turn, will burn fat. Even when you've finished exercising your body carries on burning calories at a higher rate for up to five hours – now that is something to think about!

26. Use smaller crockery.
Try to eat all your meals on smaller plates or out of smaller bowls. There is the saying "Your eyes are bigger than your belly". I think that really sums it up for me. Portion control over what I eat is a really good tool and it's something I'll always use now, as it helps me think about how much I should really be eating. It helps me roughly measure my portions without having to be obsessed with it. I believe one of the main factors in losing weight is portion control – we all tell ourselves we actually need to eat more than we really do need!

27. Go nuts.
Sensibly snacking on mixed nuts. Nuts are very nutritious for you and may actually help lower your cholesterol, but be careful not to eat too many though, because they do have lots of hidden calories in them. I measure mine out by placing some in the palm of my hand – for me, that is a portion.

28. Clever foods.
Some foods actually burn off calories whilst you're eating them, through digestion and absorption. They're called negative calories and are found in broccoli, apples, kiwis, leeks, celery, strawberries, carrots and satsumas.

29. Why?
Behind every overweight person there is a story, whether they've overeaten because of stress, like me, or boredom, loneliness, anger, depression etc. You need to look at the reasons why you're doing it, and take charge and accept them so that you can start to take control back and move forward. Stop blaming it on something else other than the fact you've put it into your mouth and overeaten in the first place. Take charge!

30. Small and steady weight loss is best.
Remember, losing weight slowly means you've more chance of keeping it off in the long term. Losing too much too fast only means your weight loss is coming from water and muscle, not fat. Fat loss is best achieved when losing weight slowly.

31. Don't have much food in the house.
I know this sounds really boring, but don't stock your cupboards up to bursting point and don't be tempted to buy any calorific snacky foods, or there will always be a temptation at your fingertips.

32. Leave the car and walk.
I know it's all the little things that can make all the difference. So walking as much as you can will really help. I am such a massive fan of plain, old-fashioned walking and I lost my first 10 stone through doing exactly that. Half an hour a day can make such a difference. If, instead of taking the car every time you go out, you start walking, you can achieve that without much effort at all.

33. Take the stairs not lifts.
Same again, it's all about thinking about what you're doing and making small changes. Take the stairs instead of the lift, go the longest way round.

Don't take the short cut. This is where all your common sense comes in, so use it.

34. Eat lots of fruit and vegetables.
At meal times, eat lots of vegetables. I always eat the same as what the rest of my family are having, but just in a smaller portion size, and I always have lots of extra vegetables on the side. It's no use trying to change your life to a healthier one and then cooking different meals for all the family – this plan is a lifestyle change so it has to be made easier and it has to be manageable. As long as you keep to the rule that the main part of your meal consists of a fist size portion of whatever you've chosen, then you can add to that as many vegetables as you want. Be sensible. You can have potatoes but just limit them. I try not to eat potatoes at all, but that's just me. Any other vegetables such as carrots, broccoli, spinach, green beans, sweetcorn, cabbage, cauliflower, lettuce, peppers, cucumber, onions, spring onions, beetroot etc – it's all about what you like to eat. Eat as much fruit as you like within reason, everything has a calorie content and it's all about retraining yourself to eat less. If you're really hungry, go and get some fruit to sustain yourself between meals. I would limit yourself to just one banana a day though, but as far as other fruits are concerned have as much as you think is realistic.

35. Chew your food slowly.
This again is probably an obvious one for you, but it does work. Eat as slowly as you can and make sure you chew your food really well. This will help fill you up and make you feel much fuller, faster.

36. Healthy snacks.
Buy in a few healthy frozen meals to store in your freezer along with some healthy snacks to keep in your cupboard. This is a lifestyle change and, at times, you will feel the need for a quick snack of some kind or a rushed meal because you've no time to make anything. Having something at hand that is healthy but does the job is important. You don't need to keep a cupboard full of such things, just one carefully chosen packet from the supermarket and a couple of frozen meals will do. Always remember, they are there for emergencies only, to be eaten when you feel you have to have that fix or you've no time. Choose carefully from the supermarket and check all the calorie content as well as saturated fat content. The smaller, the better, and always remember that as you start reading food labels you will start to understand them. It is really important that you do try to understand what they mean so you know exactly what's in the food you're buying. With

healthy frozen meals, it's easy for you when you've no time but need a meal. You can just pop one of these into the oven or microwave while you're preparing some extra vegetables to have with it. Always add lots of extra vegetables to these meals because I have found that on their own, they really don't fill you up, but with added vegetables they can work really well as a one-off meal. Fill your freezer up with your own single portion healthy meals, then you won't need to buy them from the supermarket. You can even pack them with the extra vegetables, so when you are pushed for time it's all there in the freezer for you.

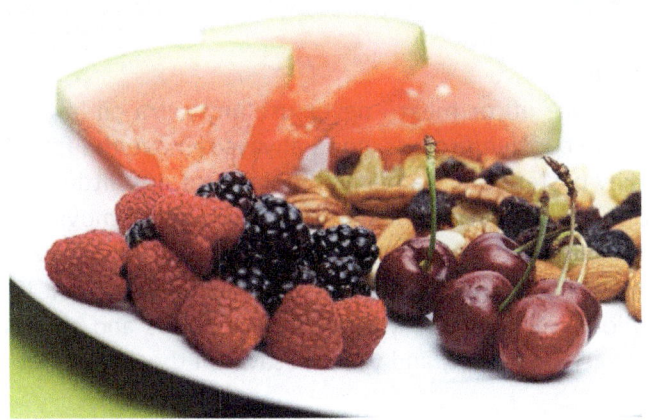

37. Don't shop when you're hungry.
This works on two levels. Shopping when you're hungry means you load your trolley up with everything your eyes take a fancy to, which often leads to you making the mistake of eating some of the things as you're loading your car up and whilst unpacking at the other end. Also you spend way too much – you're buying more than you need all because your tummy is leading the way.

38. Cooked veggies.
Whenever I cook vegetables now I make sure I cook enough for a few days or at least the next day. When they've cooled down, I pop them into a plastic container and put it into the fridge ready for the next meal. I've started having my main meal of the day at lunchtime when I can, it doesn't always work out that way, but I do try. I try to go to the gym most evenings and if I've had my tea it makes it so much harder to move and exercise on a full stomach. So having my vegetables already prepared for me to use with no need for me to start making more at lunch is a real help.

39. Feeding the family.
One of the nicest comments anyone has ever made to me was at one of Christopher's heart appointments, when his consultant, after doing all Christopher's tests and looking at his results, turned to me and said, "Well just carry on with whatever you're feeding him; whatever it is it's working because he's growing and doing really well." However large I got, that was no excuse to feed the rest of my family on gunk. We always had a full fruit bowl and ate plenty of vegetables with our meals. I didn't allow our children to eat sugary snacks or lots of takeaways. Everything I made for them always was, and still is, cooked from scratch and prepared with fresh ingredients.

40. Cooking meals.
When frying mince off or meat I never use any extra oil in the pan at the beginning of the cooking process, and I always remove the fatty liquid from it with a turkey baster before adding anything else. Just little things like that can save so many hidden calories in your food, and removing them won't make any difference to the taste. The same thing applies when making soups or sauces: I never ever fry off my vegetables in oil first. If you simply add your onions, garlic etc to your liquids in soups and sauces then you won't need to fry them first, and you will save on the extra calories and fats once again.

41. Breakfast.
Every day at breakfast I try to eat half a grapefruit before I eat anything else. I started doing it after reading an article saying that you should always eat half a grapefruit first because it help break down the fats in your food. As I always seem to eat cereal with milk for breakfast, I think it works for me, and it certainly makes sense.

42. Three meals a day.
Always try to eat three proper meals a day, or two meals and one of my smoothie replacement meals. Add small healthy snacks in between your meals too, as they keep your body moving and burning off the calories and fats throughout the day. They also keep you alert and your mind sharp, as a lack of food for long periods of time can cause headaches and sluggishness. I should know, because I had years of eating really badly and suffering in this way. Even now, if I get too busy and miss a meal by accident I eventually know because I get a headache.

43. Move.
Whatever you're doing inject movement into it. Whether it's vacuuming and dusting or just lying in the bath. I move and dance about whatever I do and it burns lots of extra calories off and you don't even know you're doing it! When I'm in the bath, I do lots of sit ups just before I get out. I can really feel my abdominal muscles working and tightening up. Also doing them in the bath is so much easier as your body is buoyant in water.

44. You are what you eat.
There was never a more true comment. I know when I've eaten something I normally wouldn't eat or drink and I don't do any extra exercise for a day or two because I feel so sluggish and bloated, and sometimes I even struggle with my bowel movement for the next day or two. At times like these I also get indigestion through the night and find sleeping difficult because it. I find it amazing that just one meal or just one day of eating too many fats and calories and no exercise can make you feel so rough; it's like suffering a food hangover, literally. There is no better feeling than feeling fit and healthy, because there really is no worse feeling then feeling sluggish and bloated. It really is worth all the effort it takes to maintain a healthy lifestyle!

45. Groups.
If you've read this book and still can't motivate yourself into making the changes you need, and you feel you can't do it on your own and that you need extra support, then there is no harm in seeking that help out for yourself. Go and talk to your doctor or join a slimming club. As long as you get the support you think you need to succeed then that's fine. For me, the diet club was never an option as I don't like the group thing and find the whole experience humiliating. I found the love and support came from my family and felt I didn't need it from anywhere else, but I appreciate that not everyone is so fortunate. I found I could achieve my new-found lifestyle on my own, and from that I went on to research and source things out for myself. I just wish there had been someone out there who had experienced it first hand, had gone through the same experiences that I have on this journey, and had written it down and documented it with good healthy family recipes for me to follow, read and make. I feel that this would have been of great inspiration and guidance for me. This is what has motivated me into putting pen to paper, so that I can try to help others who are struggling with their weight problems by offering them guidance and first-hand knowledge, along with recipes to follow. I've been through exactly the same things and have come out the other side to make a much better life for myself and my family. This is possible to do all by yourself with no fancy

diets or expensive fitness equipment – I did it and you can do it too!

46. Purge all your fat clothes.
This is great on a couple of levels. For one, it's nice to treat yourself to something new to wear after working hard to lose the weight. You don't have to replace your whole wardrobe at once, just a couple of items that you need because your old ones are slopping about. I kept a few items to remind me of where I've come from and how hard I'd worked but I certainly never want to fit into them again!

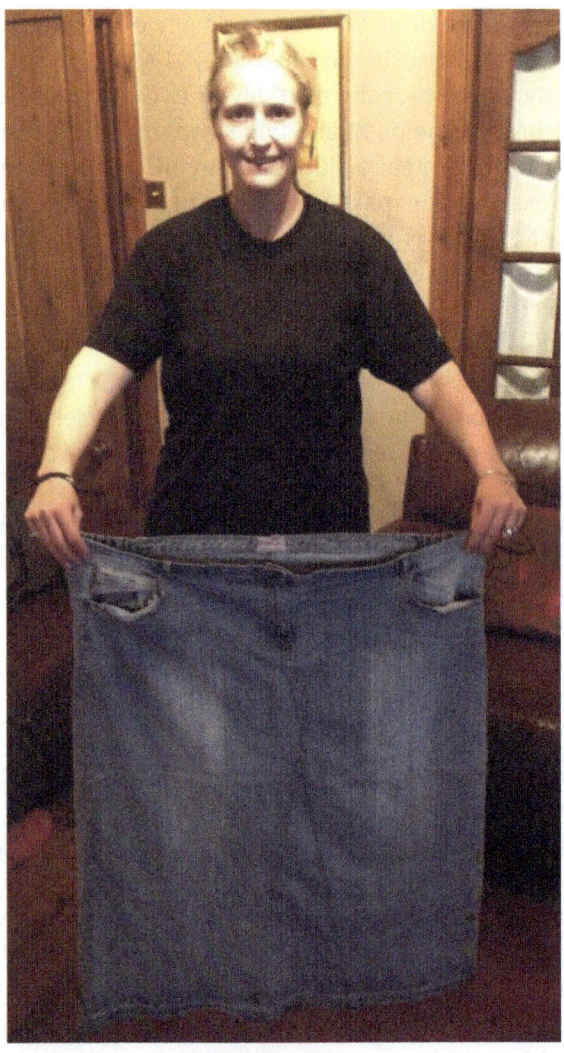

I used to wear this!

CHAPTER NINE

Your Very Own Journey!

Now it's time for you to start your very own journey.

My journey could be your journey too. All you need is to want it enough! My life today has meaning, I'm completely fulfilled in what I do and I have a purpose for the first time. I love my life and I have a very bright and healthy future, and that's all because of the journey I've been on. You too could achieve this with a little willpower and determination, which we all have and which we can all build on. Don't give me any excuses because I'm not listening!

I have been called some lovely things by some wonderful people over the last few years, such as "inspirational" and "amazing", and all because of how I've changed my life around and dealt with my problems head on, instead of burying them in the sand and carrying on comfort eating myself into an early grave. But to me it's just my life – it's not that remarkable, well, until I think back to the person I once was, that is. All this didn't happen overnight. I love the saying "All good things come to those who wait" because it's so true. I didn't put all my weight on overnight so I couldn't expect to lose it overnight either. You need to take control back and do it *now*! None of this "well when I've got back from my holidays" or "when I've got more time, I will do it". Your life is whizzing by and you need to do it now.

Okay, you need to do a little preparation, like your shopping list and planning your exercise and meals, but, realistically, how much time do you need to do all that? It's going to be tough at times but no one ever said losing weight was ever going to be easy, otherwise everyone would be skinny! In the end, only the strong will succeed.

I've been this weight for several years and I have no intention of ever regaining any of it. I go up and down within half a stone. I don't weigh often and I judge my weight by how my clothes fit me and how I feel. It's a funny thing because whenever I have checked my weight, I'm never wrong with what I feel I weigh at that moment in time. To maintain my weight I try to be very good through the week so that at weekends I can eat more or less what I want. Don't get me wrong, that doesn't mean I can totally pig out, I'm still sensible but it's my choice. I still class myself as having a food problem, or a problem with food, but I'm very aware of it. It's taken me a few years to perfect how to maintain my weight, but you do get there in the end and the benefits to your new lifestyle are immeasurable. Whether you suffer minor ailments or something more serious, once you start to make a few changes to the way you live your life, I'm quite sure that within days you'll start to feel the benefits, and long term you'll have much more energy and you'll start to look and feel much healthier. The longer you stick to my plan, the easier it gets. I didn't start losing my weight thinking I could have weekends off and eat whatever I wanted then through the week be extra good. No, I did what you have to do by being very aware of my lifestyle 24/7 until I had reached my goal.

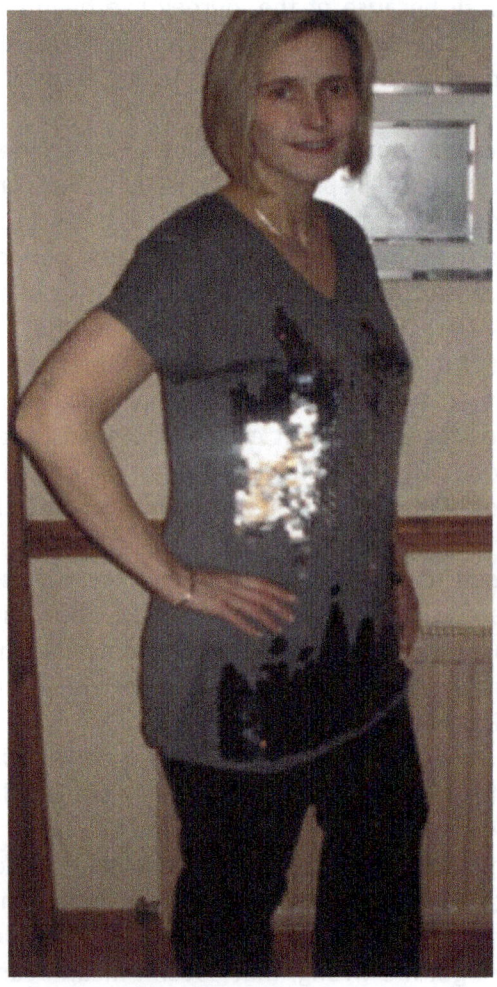

A Cautionary Word
I'd actually lost 15 stone by the time this photograph was taken, and I looked quite gaunt. I felt that I'd gone too far – it's all about finding a weight you're happy with and not being obsessed with what the scales say.

I've always loved food and always will. I'm a passionate, therapeutic baker. I love developing new and interesting healthy recipes, especially if they're cakes or puddings. I love to experiment and sample all my culinary delights. One of the biggest questions I get asked the most is, "How do I keep my weight off when I bake for a living?" Well, the answer is simply willpower. I don't believe I was born with much willpower because, if I had, I wouldn't have spent all my life being overweight. I believe I gained my willpower bit by bit, every day through my weight loss journey. It's just the same for you. You have to build up your willpower and start to believe in yourself, no one can do this for you; it has to come from you! You can do it, you really can. If you've picked up my book and read this much, then I believe you want to succeed and you're ready to make the changes necessary to do this. I believe a lot of the time we automatically talk ourselves out of these things in life, we make excuses and we fill our heads with negative thoughts instead of staying positive and true to ourselves.

One of the things I love about my life now is all the things I'm involved in through my weight loss. Before I lost my weight I would never have had the courage or confidence to go out and give talks on *Justine's Journey*, and how I've succeeded through tough, personal times in my life. I love the way people are really interested and eager to achieve a healthy, realistic lifestyle for themselves. I love motivating people and telling them about how I did it and how I saved my life and how in doing so, changed how we live as a family. There is no secret to it though, no special pill or medicine that you can take and the weight then just drops off. There are lots of diets and weight loss programmes out there but I truly believe that to achieve weight loss, and more importantly to maintain it, you have to read your body and start to understand what works for you and what motivates you. Like any addiction, at times it does get really hard and you have to fight your cravings, you then have to find that extra little bit of strength to carry on and ride those tough times. They do pass and they do get easier. I was listening to a well-known sportsman being interviewed. He summed life up and made great sense when he said that if you want to stay at top in life and achieve great things, it always takes that extra mile and there's not many people running alongside you when you do. It gets very lonely on that extra mile but that's only because a lot of people aren't willing to go that extra mile. Another good saying is: "Aim high, stay determined and you will achieve." That says it all for me really.

I used to smoke as a youngster; I gave up when I met Chris, and it was hard. But it was only hard for a certain period of time; it passed. I don't crave a cigarette any more and never have since a few weeks after giving them up. It's just the same thing with over-eating and trying to be good.

These craving pass and they then become few and far between, until the next thing you know, you've stopped your cravings altogether and you've found your routine. Meals and exercise become easier as you find out what motivates you and what makes you want to do this. As time goes by, what you initially thought would be a long time of trying to be good has gone in no time at all and that you have forgotten the old you along with the pounds you've lost in weight. In my experience, you should never start your journey by putting a timescale on it. It will take as long as it takes. It's not a competition, there's no race to the finishing line. You should just do it for yourself. For years and years I always had a particular occasion I was dieting for, whether for Christmas, for a holiday or even for my birthday. As soon as I stopped all that time-scaling, I got the whole concept of a healthy lifestyle and it worked. In the same way, I think you shouldn't really set a weight you want to particularly lose or size you want to be. Your goal should be getting fit and healthy. As you go along your journey you should work to small, manageable goals; that way, you won't feel overwhelmed with the job in hand and you'll have much more chance of achieving and maintaining your healthy lifestyle.

Don't live with regrets, life is way too short for all that nonsense. If I have one regret though, it would have to be how I lived in a very restricted way before I lost my weight. Everything was different back then and it was all self-inflicted.

All the ailments I suffered as a result of being morbidly obese have cleared up too. It really does still amaze me how many things are affected because of being overweight. Sometimes being so overweight can restrict you in taking and choosing the right exercise for you. What I say to that is: chose your exercise wisely. I'm not talking about joining a gym or going for a 10 mile run. You need to adapt your exercise and level to your own needs and keep it real! We can talk all day and make every excuse in the book about why we can't start moving, but the fact is if you really want to make these changes and lose weight then you DO have to do some form of exercise, whether that's going for a walk or sitting in a upright chair doing some sort of bog standard bicep curls with a baked bean can in each hand. The rule of thumb I always use is: if it gets you at least slightly breathless and a bit sweaty, then that's exercise. There is always something you can do as a form of exercise, just use your imagination and my "sweat" rule and it's amazing what you'll come up with. The day my journey began I went for a very short, but very sweaty walk around the block. In no time at all I had built that up to roughly two, 45 minute walks a day. I went for one in the morning, as soon as I had dropped the children off at school, and another in the evening. I didn't do that every day, just when I could fit it in to my daily routine. You should be looking at, at least 20 minutes of exercise 5 days a week, then build on that. Yes, we all have lives and things that fill our time through the day, but ask yourself the question: Do you want to do this or not? As well as eating a healthy mixed diet, including a whole range of rainbow coloured fruit and vegetables, exercising should also be at the top of your lifestyle changes list.

Okay, so you're off on your journey and everything's going really well. At this point I'm going to map out how I initially started my journey and what emotions were going through my head. I will at times talk it through as if it's your journey and how you're feeling, to enable you to feel all the emotions of what it's like to achieve a new lifestyle...

You've had a great first day and feel on top of the world, as well as really motivated to succeed and kick this thing. Day Two is a good one also, even though anything and everything foodie seems to be highlighted in your head and everywhere you look it's food, food and more food. You're starting to pee more too and never seem to be off the loo – that's your system flushing itself out and will settle down. We're still in the zone, we can kick this, hell yeah baby! Days Four and Five and the pressure is on, you're starting to crave anything you would normally class as a treat. You're starting to feel quite tired and drained. You're even starting feel cold even though it's quite warm outside. Your head is doing itself in with the thought of how you are going to have to be good for the rest of your life, all this effort and you don't even look or feel any slimmer. Depressing! At this point, I tried to drink extra water or low calorie cordial all day and I was even known to sneak off and sleep for a couple of hours through the day once or twice in the coming weeks, just to get out of this miserable, hungry, bored feeling I had and what I can only describe as "detoxing hell". If I crack now I'll be back to square one and why am I doing this? I want to live! I want to see my children and their children grow up!

Day Six is a slightly more positive day and you're managing quite well even though you're still very cold and every image in your head involves some kind of food. The walking for exercise is getting easier and giving you something to focus on, and it even makes you feel like you're not wasting all your time walking then shovelling crap down your throat. Exercising is giving you even more incentive to stay on track.

Week Two gets slightly more manageable even though you've experienced a few ups and downs and you're very snappy with the family at the slightest thing. It's a bit like having your period emotionally (if you're a woman) without having a period. You're still having to fight some cravings but, because you're filling up on regular healthy meals, the craving are becoming less and more manageable.

Week Three is a breeze and you'll wish you'd felt like this from the very start. You're the king or queen of the world and you WILL succeed! Walking for exercise is really easy, and mentally you're feeling great and not as tired and drained.

But Week Four is pretty hard. It has plenty of downs and you're having to dig deep to keep motivated. At this stage, I was quite overwhelmed that I had just passed a milestone in my life – I'd never stayed so focussed for so long and I could literally feel the weight dropping off me, even though no one could tell yet. No one has mentioned that you are looking slimmer, but these things will take time. You're not focussing on the amount of weight, more the small healthy goals and that's what's keeping you going at this present moment. To be fair, like all the diets I'd been on previously, this one was no different from the perspective that I hadn't told anyone what I was doing. *Not even family and close friends*, as I was so worried about not succeeding and looking like a complete failure. A failure is not what you want to be, so you're focussing hard on the thought of what people will say when they can tell you've lost weight. In your head all the time is the thought that you want to survive and live for your family. You're so going to do this; failure is NOT an option. It's been four whole weeks since you've changed your lifestyle and you've lost a considerable amount of weight. At this stage, I didn't know that I would go on to lose another 12 stone in weight, and unfortunately for me, still no one had noticed me losing weight and looking slimmer. That was okay though, I was doing this for me and my family, not to just look better.

Week Five and you can see the sun at the end of the rainbow now and things seems so much easier and more manageable. You've got into such a natural easy routine. You plan meals a day or so in advance, and you just accept you're walking for your exercise if that's the exercise you have chosen to do. You don't feel as red and sweaty any more when exercising like you once did, so you must be getting slightly fitter too. I had to dig out old clothes that hadn't fitted me for years, some of them weren't even fashionable but I had to wear something. No way would I buy new clothes at this stage. You're now very determined to go a lot smaller in your size of clothes so buying all new stuff at this stage would be a complete waste of money.

Week Six will always stay with me as being a pinnacle one, a real turning point for me. It was when my lifestyle change became a way of life for me and it all just clicked into place. No longer was it a chore. It was just how the new me rolled along! It certainly wasn't and didn't feel like a diet any more and I'd even stopped thinking about food all the time. Then a close friend asked if I'd lost some weight and went on to say I was looking good – Hallelujah! What a moment that was and such an uplifting thing to hear. At that stage I had no idea that the compliments would keep coming thick and fast over the next five years!

That was a sample timeline over the first six weeks of my journey and what could be your journey too. Some of the things you'll experience will be easier to cope with or perhaps harder to cope with than I found. I didn't sugar coat any of it as I tried to remember some of the hardest moments and things I went through. Everyone will experience their own ups and downs. I just wanted to get across the fact that it's harder at some points than others and for me, after the first six weeks of my journey, it began to feel like a way of life and manageable, just like it does for me today. No chore, no hard struggles, just a routine where my old habits have disappeared along with my weight. To me, life's all about habits, good or bad ones. Through changing my sloppy, bad eating habits I regained a healthy lifestyle and I'm now living it for the first time in my life.

It really is that simple and achievable.

Will your journey start today?

I know how you are feeling; I've felt like that too. I know how much better you will feel in a very short time – it's how I feel every single day and it feels fantastic!

Now you are ready to start your very own journey…

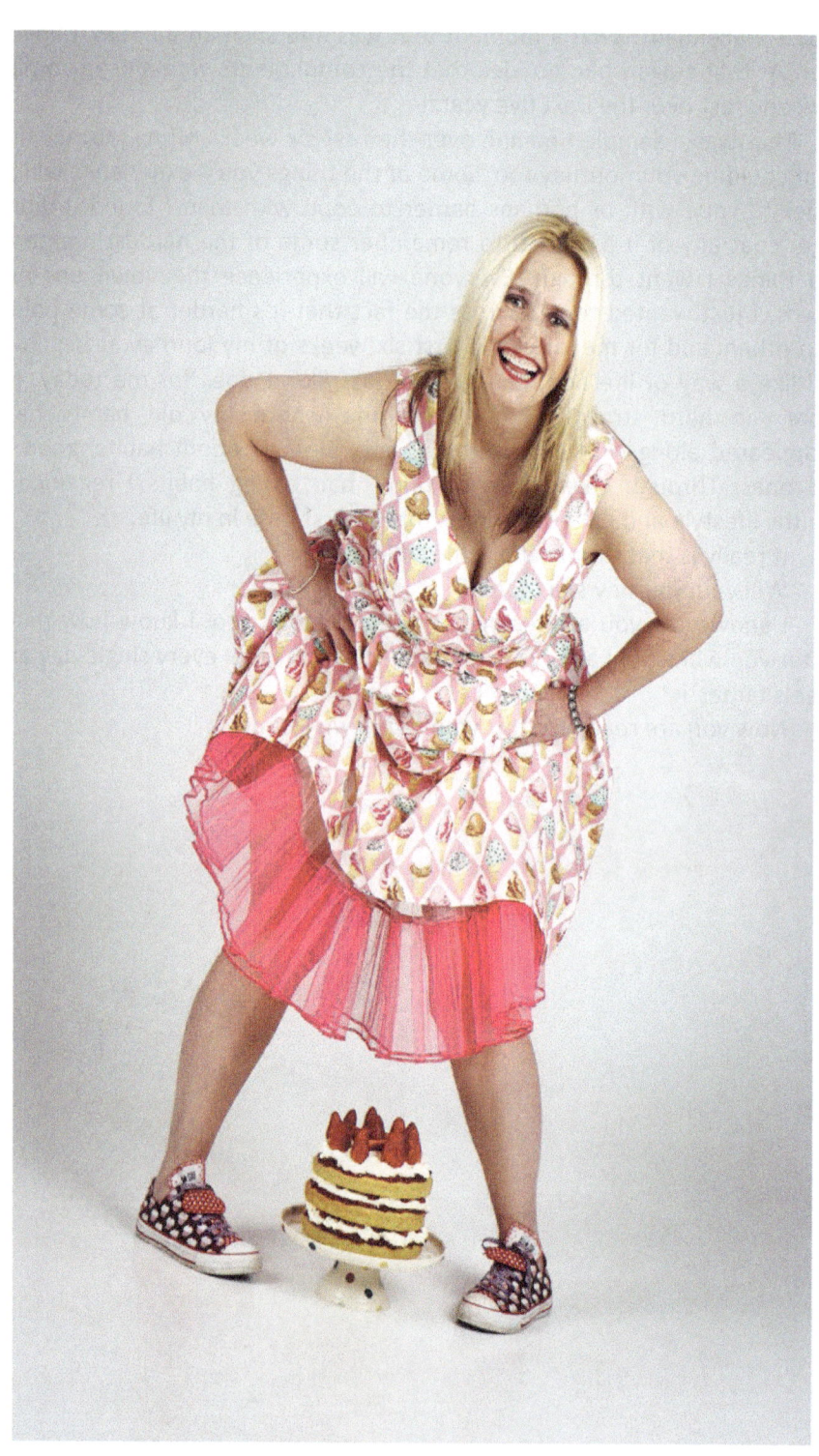

CHAPTER 10

Breakfasts

Choose one of the following for breakfast every morning.

- Bran flakes with skimmed milk and a handful of sultanas. I make this and cover with cling film until I'm ready to eat it. It thickens up and isn't as crunchy – just the way I like it.

- One fruit scone cut in half with one dessertspoon of jam. This doesn't seem a lot or even look a lot when it's on your plate, but it does fill you up and is a sweet change in the morning.

- One poached egg on one slice of dry toasted wholemeal bread. This also doesn't look that much but the egg is slow releasing, so it does fill you up and keeps you going until the next meal. If you struggle making poached egg here's some tips. Use a round saucepan, boil the water and add a good slug of vinegar. With the water still boiling, stir it around, then drop in your egg so it swirls around in a circular motion. After about a minute turn the heat off and leave your egg for another 60 seconds. Remove from pan with a slotted spoon. You should now have a lovely softly poached runny in the middle egg. If all that is too much first thing in the morning, another way to poach your egg is to place it into a plastic microwave container, knife the yolk and cover with a lid, cook in the microwave until it's done – even my children can do poached eggs like this.

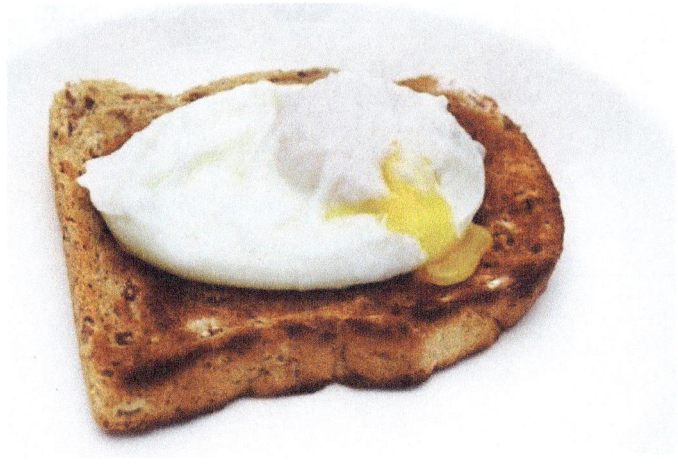

- Porridge and honey. Place one small cupful of porridge oats in a saucepan or microwave jug, add one cup full of skimmed milk and one cupful of water. Cook in your pan or in the microwave until the oats have thickened and there's no liquid left. This usually takes about 3 to 5 minutes. If you like it quite runny add more boiling water. When it's done, place in your breakfast bowl and add a teaspoon of honey; not only will honey sweeten the oats up and make it taste nice, it is also very good for you. Eating porridge for breakfast is a very good way of keeping hunger at bay until your next meal, as the oats are also slow releasing and they keep you feeling full.

- Fruit and yogurt. Into your bowl place some mixed fruits, i.e. strawberries, blueberries, raspberries, a cut up apple etc. I tend to keep away from bananas as I like to have a banana on its own later in the day to give me that boost of energy when I'm flagging in the afternoon. Over the top of your fruit spoon a teaspoonful of runny honey and 3 dessertspoons full of low fat natural yogurt. I then sprinkle on top one dessertspoon full of grape nuts (you can find them in the cereal section of any good supermarket). Grape nuts contain whole grain wheat flour, which is high in dietary fibre and is an excellent source of folic acid and iron. Or you could use a spoonful of muesli instead. I sometimes make a smaller version of this as my pudding after my tea in the evening.

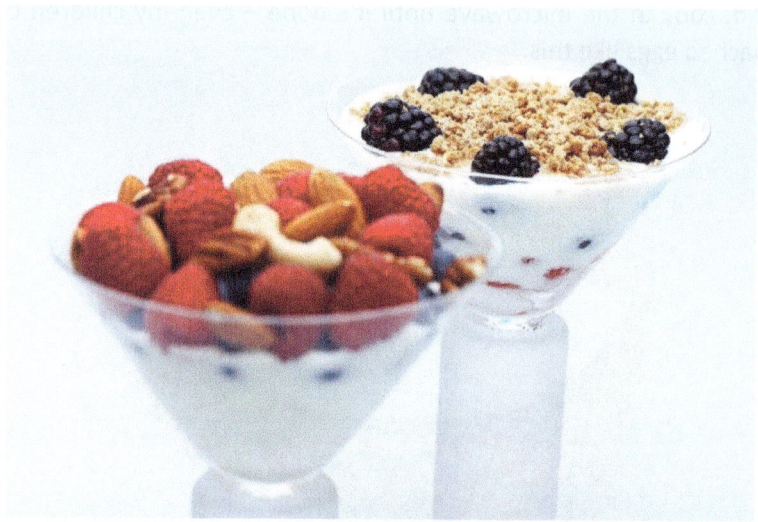

CHAPTER 11

Light Lunches

This chapter gives you the healthy lunch options I ate after the first six months of sticking to having one of my nutritious smoothies for lunch (see Chapter Fifteen) when I first started my weight loss journey. I still continue to eat these healthy lunch options below to maintain my weight.

EGG PITTA

This makes a very quick and chunky alternative to a sandwich. Eggs are also very good for being healthy, as they're slow releasing and fill you up for longer – just what you need!

Serves 1
1 hard boiled egg, chopped
1 dessertspoon of low fat mayonnaise
A little red onion, peeled and chopped – optional
A little lettuce, washed and shredded – optional
1 tomato, sliced
1 regular size brown pitta bread
Salt/pepper to taste

1. Combine the egg, salt and mayonnaise together.

2. Carefully split open the pitta bread and add the lettuce and onion if you're using them.

3. Fill the pitta with the egg mayonnaise mixture.

4. You can make this beforehand and wrap it up in cling film. It also travels well.

SPICY PORK BURGER

Sometimes I feel like tucking into a meaty burger and this one is the nicest low calorie one I've found. If you want to make it even more healthy, eat it in a brown bun or even on its own just with vegetables.

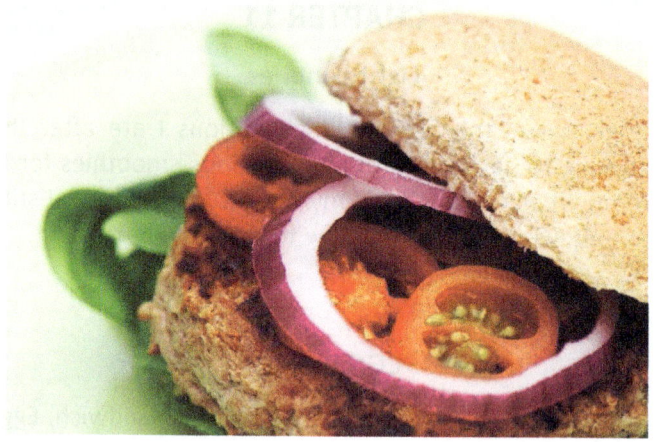

Makes approximately 8
1 500g packet of lean minced pork
2 heaped teaspoons of cumin
2 heaped teaspoons coriander
2 heaped teaspoons chilli powder
1 finely chopped onion
4 cloves of garlic

1. Place the pork and all the spices into a large mixing bowl. With clean hands mix everything together – really get stuck in. My children usually do this job for me and they thoroughly enjoy it.

2. Add the finely chopped onion to this, then peel and finely chop the garlic and add to the mixture.

3. Mix everything together really well with your hands and divide into patty size balls. Pat each one down to make the shape of a burger.

4. Place in the fridge for at least half an hour so that when you cook them they stay in shape and don't fall apart. You can do this in advance and at this stage freeze some on a flat baking tray. Once frozen, remove them from the baking tray and bag up and place back into the freezer ready for another day.

5. I either grill these or place on a greased baking tray and cook in the oven for approximately 20 minutes on 200C/400F/Gas mark 6. You can pan fry these, but you will need to add extra oil to the pan before frying, so for me and my family frying is not an option.

HEALTHY HOUMOUS

I love houmous; a world without houmous would be truly awful. Houmous has to be one of my all time favourite foods, any variety will do. Years ago I used to buy it until I found out it was easy to make at home and also very inexpensive, much cheaper than buying ready-made. For quickness, you can use tinned chickpeas. Try boiling up dried ones, they're even cheaper. I do not add any oil to any of my houmous recipes and personally can't tell the difference without. Instead, I use water or lemon juice for an even healthier option. All my different houmous keep well, for up to 2 weeks stored in airtight containers in the fridge.

Spinach and Garlic Houmous

1 tin of chickpeas
2 cloves of garlic
2 teaspoons cumin
2 large handfuls fresh spinach leaves
Splash of lemon juice
Splash of water
Salt and pepper to taste

Place all the above ingredients into a food processor apart from the water and whiz together until it is all stuck to the sides. Scrape back from the sides and add a splash of water. Whiz together again. If it's still a bit too thick add a little more water and whiz again; if not, it's done. As easy as that! I serve on brown pitta bread topped off with red onions and cherry tomatoes.

Sweet Chilli Houmous

1 tin of chickpeas or the same amount approximately in dried ones that have been cooked to their packet instructions
1 fresh red chilli, deseeded
1 dessertspoon of sweet chilli sauce from a jar (any good supermarket will sell it)
2 cloves garlic, peeled and chopped
Splash lemon juice
Splash of water
Salt and pepper to taste

1. Place all the above ingredients into a food processor and blitz together until they're combined.

2. Scrap back from the sides of the processor bowl and if needed, add a splash of water – be careful not to add too much though – and whiz again.

That's it! Serve as before on a toasted brown pitta topped off with cherry tomatoes and red onion.

Roasted Red Pepper Houmous

This one my friend, Cath, makes which is absolutely delicious, yummy.

1 tin of chickpeas
2 clove of garlic, peeled and chopped
1 red pepper, deseeded, peeled and chopped roughly into 4 pieces
Splash lemon juice
Splash water
Salt and pepper to taste

1. In a roasting tin place the chopped red pepper. Roast in a pre-heated oven on 220C for 10 minutes or until it has collapsed and gone soft.

2. Place all the above including the red peppers but not the water into a food processor and blitz until well mixed. Scrape back from the sides of your processor and add a little water if it's needed, and blitz again.

Serve as before. Enjoy!

Roasted Red Onion Houmous

This recipe again is my friend Cath's, who most generously shared it with me because we are both Houmous Heads, as I call us.

1 tin of chickpeas
1 large red onion, peeled and chopped
2 cloves of garlic, peeled and chopped
Splash of lemon juice
Splash of water
Salt and pepper to taste

1. Place the onion in the oven for 30 minutes on about 200C.

2. When the onion is cooked, add it to your food processor along with all the other ingredients apart from the water and blitz until everything is well mixed.

3. Scrape back from the sides and add water if needed.

4. Serve as before.

My Plain Old Houmous

This one is the same as all the others but with no added extra flavours from other ingredients, but it tastes just as good and is very easy to make, and moreish.

1 tin of chickpeas
2 cloves of garlic, peeled and chopped
Splash of lemon juice
Splash of water
Salt and pepper to taste

1. Same as all the rest: blitz together all the above ingredients apart from the water. Scrape back from the sides of your food processor, add a little water and blitz again.

2. Serve on a toasted brown pitta bread or just use as a dip to have with carrots and other vegetables.

SMOKED MACKEREL PATE

This is great on toast, crusty bread or the healthier option of brown pitta bread or Ryvitas. It's very easy to make and tastes wonderful. This snack hits the spot for me for a light lunch or for tea with a side salad. You can also serve this as a starter. Either way, it's a Winner! Excuse the pun.

1 packet mackerel fillets, about 4 to a packet
Half a tub of low fat cream cheese
1 dessertspoon crème fraiche/natural Greek yogurt
Splash of lemon juice
Salt/pepper

1. Take all the skin off the mackerel fillets and mash flesh well with a fork.

2. Add the rest of the ingredients and mix well.

3. Serve on crusty bread or toasted brown pitta bread.

This pate keeps for up to a week in an airtight container in the fridge.

PITTA PIZZA

These are very, very tasty indeedy. You can eat these as a canapé or as a lunch option. You can add what you like, so please experiment with them. They are healthy especially if you use as little cheese on the top as possible. Why not try using edam or goats cheese for an even more healthier option. When I make these my three children love to join in and make their own. It's a great family hands-on making thing and it's also great to teach children about different foods and tastes.

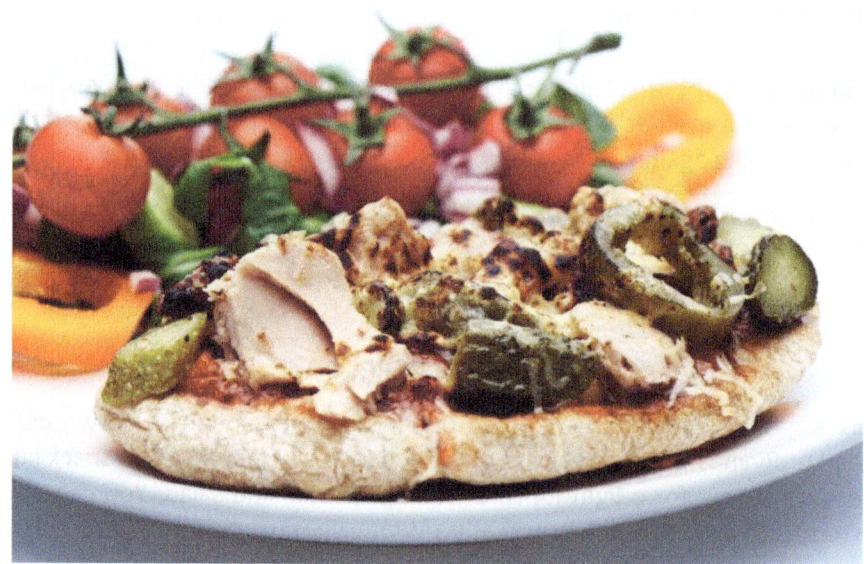

For the tomato topping

2 tins chopped tomatoes
Squirt of tomato ketchup
Slug of Worcestershire sauce
4 cloves of garlic, peeled and finely chopped
1 dessertspoon dried Italian seasoning

1. Drain the tinned tomatoes and place in a bowl. Add the rest of the ingredients and mix well, tasting to see if you need more Worcestershire sauce.

This lasts for weeks in an airtight container in the fridge; in actual fact, it gets better with age.

Topping for the pizza – mix and match what you like

Capers
Mushrooms
Olives
Red onion
Peppers
Sun dried tomatoes
Tinned tuna in brine
Ham
German sausage
A good strong cheese (stilton or gorgonzola, or for a healthier option try edam or goats cheese)
A packet of brown pitta breads

1. Place pittas on a baking tray and top with the tomato sauce mix. Add the toppings you like and finish off with some grated cheese.

2. Place in a hot oven approximately 220C for roughly 10 minutes or until the cheese has turned golden brown. Enjoy!

CHAPTER 12
Healthy Teas
CORONATION CHICKEN

This little recipe gem is one of my personal favourites. It's so versatile, you can eat it on a jacket potato, with a mixed salad or even in a sandwich. The only trouble with it is you can't ever seem to make enough! Every time I make an airtight container full for the fridge in come all the family to eat forkfuls. I think they must be able smell the stuff being made.

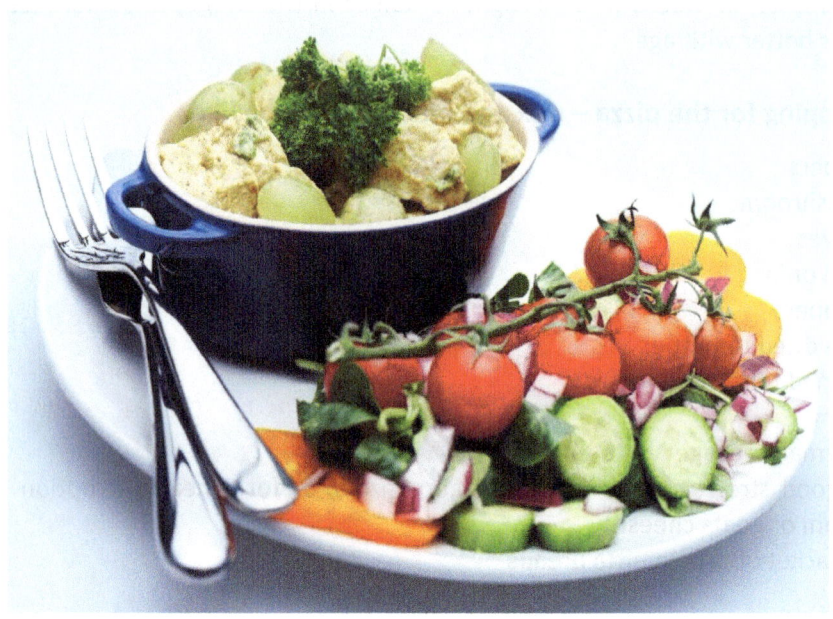

Serves 4
4 skinless chicken breast fillets, cooked
8oz/225g low fat fromage frais
1 tablespoon medium curry powder
2 tablespoons mango chutney
8oz/225g seedless green grapes, halved
Good splash lemon juice
1 tablespoon fresh/dried parsley – optional
Salt/pepper

1. Roughly dice the cooked chicken fillets into cubes and place in a mixing bowl.

2. In another mixing bowl combine the fromage frais, curry powder, lemon juice, mango chutney and parsley.

3. Cut the grapes into halves, add to the cubed chicken and mix. Then add all the fromage frais mixture and combine well. Season to taste.

4. Keep in an airtight container in the fridge until ready to serve.

Serving suggestions: big mixed salad, or a jacket potato, or in a granary bread sandwich.

MOUSSAKA

This is also a very good winter warmer that all the family can sit around the table and eat together. You can either serve with extra seasonal vegetables or a mixed salad. This serves at least four big portions – more than enough for leftovers.

Serves at least 4
1 onion
500g lean mince meat
Large tin chopped tomatoes
1 beef stock cube
2 courgettes
3 large white potatoes
300g low fat Greek yogurt
2 eggs
A handful of grated cheese (cheddar, edam – anything you have in the fridge)
A big slug of Worcestershire sauce

1. Preheat the oven to 200C/400F/Gas mark 6. Finely peel and chop the onion. Place in a pan over the hob and fry off with the mince until browned, stirring regularly.

2. Add the tinned tomatoes and crumble in the stock cube. Add the Worcestershire sauce and turn the heat down to low. Simmer for approximately 10 minutes.

3. Peel and thinly slice the potatoes and par-boil for 5 minutes and then drain. Slice the courgettes. Place the mince mixture into a large ovenproof dish approximately 9in x 7in. Top with the sliced courgettes and then the potatoes.

4. Whisk together the yogurt and eggs until smooth. Pour over the top of the potatoes and sprinkle with the grated cheese.

5. Cook in the oven for approximately 30–40 minutes until golden brown on top and bubbling.

SPICED SUGAR ROASTED SALMON ON A BED OF CABBAGE

I love fish and we try to eat it as much as possible, so finding a new recipe to cook different types of fish is always good for a change. This recipe is quite sweet but we like it. It's also another very simple dish to make.

Serves 4
4 salmon fillets
1oz/30g soft brown sugar
½ teaspoon ground cinnamon
1 green cabbage
Salt/pepper

1. Place the salmon fillets on a baking tray. Mix together the sugar and cinnamon. Divide between the four pieces of salmon, rubbing all over until they are evenly coated.

2. Leave for half an hour until some of the moisture has come out of the salmon.

3. Finely slice the cabbage and wash it.

4. Heat the grill. Place the salmon fillets under a medium grill for about 7–10 minutes until cooked. The salmon should look opaque and flake easily.

5. Steam the cabbage for a few minutes in a steamer, until it's just cooked.

6. Season really well with salt and lots of freshly ground pepper. Divide the cabbage between four plates. Serve the salmon on top and add boiled new potatoes on the side.

VEGETABLE KEDGEREE

Packed with colourful vegetables, this speedy kedgeree gives you a healthy boost just by looking at it. It's very easy to make too.

Serves 4
1 onion, peeled and sliced
1 red pepper, deseeded and sliced
1 carrot, peeled and chopped
1 courgette, chopped
3½oz/100g trimmed green beans
Small tin sweetcorn
9oz/250g pack of express pilau rice (already cooked)
2oz/50g feta cheese

1. Finely peel and chop the onion and carrot, de-seed and dice the red pepper and cube the courgette. In a large frying pan, dry fry all the vegetables until softened.

2. Cut the beans in half and drain the sweetcorn. Add along with the rice to the other vegetables and fry also.

3. Cook for a further 5 minutes on a very low heat and then crumble in the feta cheese, stir and serve immediately.

LIVER, CHIPOLATA SAUSAGE AND BEAN CASSEROLE

This is one recipe I've been making all my married life. It's one of our favourites. Once you've browned off the sausages you can also pop this into a slow cooker and leave to cook until ready to serve.

Serves 4
4oz/110g low fat chipolata sausages
12oz/350g lambs liver, sliced thinly
1 onion, peeled and sliced
1 tin of low calorie tomato soup
2 teaspoons Worcestershire sauce
1 teaspoon white wine vinegar
1 teaspoon Dijon mustard
1 large tin low calorie baked beans

1. Grill the sausages and leave to one side.

2. Place the liver in an ovenproof dish (or into a slow cooker, if using), along with the sausages and peeled and sliced onion.

3. Mix the rest of the ingredients together and pour over the liver and sausages.

4. Cover with a lid and pop in the oven for 45 minutes on 180C/350F/Gas mark 4 or if using a slow cooker, leave on low all day.

5. Serve with lots of extra vegetables on the side.

PORK PAPRIKA

The paprika, onion and yogurt add an exotic touch to these delicious pork chops.

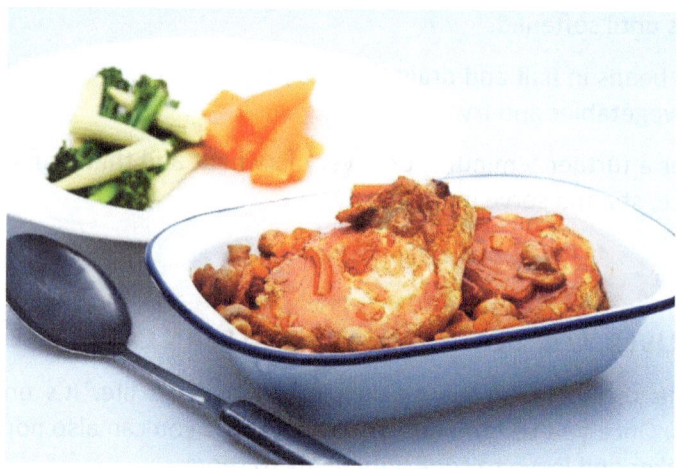

Serves 4
4 lean boneless pork chops
1 onion, peeled diced
½ tablespoon oil
1 tablespoon paprika
2oz/50g tomato puree
125ml boiling water with 1 chicken stock cube added
6oz/175g small button mushrooms, sliced
10oz/275g low fat natural yogurt

1. Pre-heat oven to 180C/350F/Gas mark 4.

2. Season pork chops and put under the grill to seal on both sides. Remove from the grill and discard any fat. Place chops to one side.

3. In a flameproof casserole pan, place the oil and add the peeled and finely chopped onions. After they have softened and browned add the paprika and blend in. Add the tomato puree and mix through. Remove from the heat and stir in the stock.

4. Return to the heat and bring to the boil, stirring all the time. Taste and season at this stage. Add the pork chops. Cover with the lid, and place in the pre-heated oven for 30 minutes.

5. Five minutes before the end of cooking, remove from the oven and add the mushrooms, place back into the oven. Just before serving, spoon over the yogurt. Serve with seasonal vegetables.

THAI CHILLI CHICKEN ON A BED OF BROWN RICE

I love any recipe which includes brown rice, I love the stuff and it always makes me feel super healthy after I've eaten it. Before you start making this dish, it's always advisable to marinade the chicken the night before or at least in the morning of the day you're going to be cooking it. The chicken will be much more tender and the flavours will have really soaked into it.

Serves 4
2 garlic cloves, peeled and crushed
1 lemongrass stalk, finely chopped
1 tablespoon grated fresh ginger
1 red chilli, deseeded and chopped
2 tablespoons chopped coriander
4 tablespoons lime juice
1 tablespoon soy sauce
350g skinless chicken breasts, sliced into strips
300g brown rice
1 dessertspoon of olive oil
4 shallots, peeled and thinly sliced
1 medium carrot, peeled and cut into strips
3½oz/100g sugar snap peas or mangetout, cut into halves
2 pak choi heads, roughly shredded

1. In a large mixing bowl add the garlic, lemongrass, ginger, chilli, coriander, lime juice and soy sauce. Add the chicken, mix well and cover for at least 30 minutes, or more if you have time.

2. When you're ready to eat, cook the brown rice in lightly salted boiling water, following the packet instructions.

3. Ten minutes before the rice is ready, heat the olive oil in a wok or large frying pan. Lift chicken out of the marinade juices and stir-fry for 5–6 minutes. Then add the shallots, carrots and sugar snap peas or mangetout. Stir fry for a further 2–3 minutes then add the pak choi and all the marinade juices. Cook until the pak choi has wilted, about 2 more minutes.

4. Drain the brown rice and serve alongside the chilli chicken.

WALDORF SALAD

Traditionally, Waldorf salad contains apples, celery, high fat walnuts and an even higher fat mayonnaise. Here, instead, I've made a very tasty low fat version which also looks deliciously creamy.

Serves 4
2 apples
2 dessertspoons lemon juice
4 sticks of celery, washed and sliced
6 spring onions, washed and finely sliced
1 large tin of butterbeans, drained and rinsed
1 tablespoon chopped parsley
Salt/pepper

For the dressing

6oz/175g low fat fromage frais
2 tablespoons white wine vinegar
1 tablespoon lemon juice
¼ teaspoon ground turmeric
2 teaspoons white sugar
Salt/pepper to taste

1. Quarter and core the apples, then cut and cube them. Place in a bowl and add the lemon juice.

2. Add the celery and spring onions. Mix in the butterbeans and parsley, season well.

3. In another bowl mix together all the dressing ingredients until everything is combined well.

4. Pour the dressing over the prepared apple, celery and spring onion, and toss.

5. Serve on a bed of mixed lettuce.

This also goes really well with cooked cold meat or smoked fish.

PORK RAGOUT

For a change I do enjoy a little bit of pork. This recipe is another easy, cheap and cheerful example of how healthy cooking can be quick and simple, and much better for you.

Serves 4
1 clove garlic, peeled and crushed
1lb/450g lean pork fillet, trimmed and cubed
3½oz/100g button mushrooms
6oz/175g courgettes cut into julienne strips (matchstick size pieces)
1 green pepper, deseeded and cut into strips
1 large tin chopped tomatoes
1 onion
¼ pint/150ml beef stock (or boiling water with 2 added beef stock cubes)
1 tablespoon chopped fresh basil
Salt/pepper

1. Dry fry the pork, garlic, onion and mushrooms in a non-stick frying pan for a couple of minutes or until the pork is browned and the onions are translucent.

2. Add the vegetables, beef stock, tinned tomatoes, basil and season well.

3. Bring to the boil, then turn the heat down and simmer for 40–45 minutes.

4. If necessary, remove the lid towards the end of cooking so the sauce can reduce down and thicken slightly.

5. Serve on its own or, if you're feeling extra hungry, you could have it with some additional steamed vegetables or some steamed brown rice.

SPICY CHICKPEA CASSEROLE

You certainly don't need to be a vegetarian to enjoy a non-meat dish like this one. I sometimes eat this for my lunch too – well, that's when I'm feeling I need a little more nourishment after one of my long runs. I usually double the quantity of all the ingredients in this dish and keep the leftovers in an airtight container in the fridge so it's at hand to have straight away when I don't feel like cooking. It also freezes well too.

Serves 4
1 large tin of chickpeas, washed and drained
1 onion, peeled and diced
1 large tin chopped tomatoes
2 vegetables stock cubes
½ teaspoon ground coriander
2 heaped teaspoons cumin
½ teaspoon chilli powder
8oz/225g dry weight of brown rice
8oz/225g mushrooms, sliced
1 tablespoon chopped fresh coriander
Salt/pepper

1. In a large lidded pan add all the ingredients apart from the brown rice and fresh coriander. Give it a good old stir and bring to the boil. Turn down and simmer for 8–10 minutes. Season to taste.

2. Cook the brown rice as instructed on the packet.

3. When everything's finished cooking, add the chopped coriander to the chickpeas and stir.

4. Serve the spicy chickpeas on a bed of brown rice.

Now, how quick and easy is that!

TUNA STUFFED BEEF TOMATOES

This is a great meal if you're not wanting to eat much and you fancy being extra good and keeping it light. This meal is primarily cooked in a microwave but can also be baked in the oven. Very, very simple again but packed with plenty of flavours. See, who said healthy cooking was boring and flavourless?

Serves 2
2 large beef tomatoes (if you can't find any, go for the largest tomatoes you can find)
1 small tin of tuna in brine, drained and mashed
½ onion, peeled and finely chopped
½ small tin sweetcorn
2oz/50g edam cheese, grated
Salt/pepper

1. Slice the tomatoes in half and scoop out all the insides into a bowl.

2. Fork or mash the pulp and add the rest of the ingredients apart from the cheese.

3. Fill the tomatoes halves back up with the tomato pulp mixture.

4. Grate the cheese and sprinkle on top of all four tomato halves.

5. Place in the microwave for approximately 3 minutes depending on the wattage of your microwave. Alternatively, you can pop them onto a baking tray and place in a pre-heated oven on about 200C for 8–10 minutes, or until the cheese is all bubbly and brown on top.

6. Serve with either a mixed salad or extra steamed vegetables.

SPICED LAMB WITH COUSCOUS

This dish is packed with flavour and, considering it's a healthy dish with fewer calories, is a pretty good healthy option. A well cooked lamb dish is heaven to me. I love the flavour and texture of a spicy lamb dish where the meat is really tender. Hope you enjoy this dish as much as my family and I do.

Serves 2
8oz/225g lean lamb steak, diced
1 onion, peeled and chopped
1 clove of garlic, peeled and crushed
½ teaspoon ground cumin
2oz/50g dried apricot, diced
¼ pint/150ml stock (fresh chicken, lamb or vegetable stock or made with a stock cube)
4oz/110g dry weight couscous
1 tablespoon fresh chopped mint

1. In a large non-stick pan, dry fry the lamb, onion and garlic until the meat is browned.

2. Add the cumin, apricots and stock. Season to taste and bring to the boil. Turn down low and simmer uncovered for approximately 15–20 minutes.

3. Meanwhile, make the couscous according to the packet instructions.

4. Stir the mint into the couscous then add all this to the pan of lamb and stir well.

5. Cover with a lid and carry on simmering for a further 8–10 minutes or until the lamb is tender. Add more stock if needed.

6. Serve with lots of extra steamed vegetables.

SHEPHERD'S PIE

This is a great tea-time meal. I've never followed a particular recipe for this, this is just how I've always made it. It's very, very tasty indeedy with plenty of flavours.

500g pack of minced lamb
1.5kg white potatoes (any mashing potatoes are good, e.g. Maris Piper)
1 onion, peeled and sliced
3 cloves garlic, peeled and crushed
6 mushrooms, sliced
1 dessertspoon mint sauce
1 dessertspoon beef gravy granules
3 big slugs Worcestershire sauce
2 medium size carrots, peeled, cut into very small squares and blanched for 4 minutes OR 2 handfuls of frozen peas
1 dessertspoon margarine
A little milk
A small piece of cheddar cheese, grated
Dried mint
Salt/pepper

1. Pre-heat the oven to 200C or equivalent. In a large pan fry off the minced lamb (do not use any extra oil, the lamb has enough in it). Add the onions, garlic and mushrooms and brown for 5 minutes, stirring continuously. With a large spoon remove some of the fat that's come off the meat and discard.

2. Turn the heat down and add a splash of water, gravy granules, Worcestershire sauce, mint sauce, blanched carrots or garden peas and season well. Cover with a lid and simmer for about 8–10 minutes. At this stage, if it's too thick add another splash of water.

3. Peel and cube the potatoes and in a large pan of water bring them to the boil. Turn the heat down and simmer for 10 minutes or until a sharp knife falls from the centre of a potato when you test it.

4. Remove the potatoes from the heat and drain. Either with a masher, potato ricer or an electric hand mixer, start to mash the potatoes, adding the margarine and then a splash of milk until they're nice and creamy. Season to taste.

5. Add the meat mixture to a large casserole or lasagne dish and spread out evenly along the bottom. Carefully top off with the mashed potatoes, smoothing out with a fork as you go. Finally, sprinkle with grated cheddar cheese and some dried mint.

6. Place in the oven for 40–45 minutes or until the cheese has turned golden brown and the whole dish is bubbling away nicely.

7. Serve with lots of extra steamed vegetables.

PAELLA

This is my take on the Spanish dish of paella. It makes a quick tea-time meal for all the family. You can use any fish in it, it's up to you. I'll list what I use and you can leave out or add what you want. It's a very tasty meal with all the fish and that makes it very healthy too. This dish is my ickle boy, Christopher's very favourite, so we have this quite often. It takes about 30 minutes to make from start to finish including prepping time.

This feeds a family of 5
1 splash of olive oil
300g paella rice
2½–3 pints of boiling water
3 fish/vegetable or chicken stock cubes
3 teaspoons paprika
2 handfuls of frozen peas
2 skinless chicken breasts, cubed
1 onion, peeled and sliced
3 cloves of garlic, peeled and crushed

Fish: I buy a pre-packed fish mix from the supermarket. You could ask your fishmonger for a mix of fish off cuts or buy some of the following fish separately: cod, smoked haddock, salmon, mussels, squid, raw tiger prawns, lobster, cockles etc.

1. Start by cubing up the chicken and frying it off in the olive oil. I always use a heavy bottomed cast iron pan for this. Add the onions and garlic, this should take about 5 minutes or until the chicken is sealed and the onions/garlic translucent.

2. Add the rice and paprika and stir until the rice is fully coated with the paprika.

3. Add the water, stock cubes and frozen peas, give it a good stir and season well.

4. Leave to cook on a high simmer for about 20 minutes or until the rice has taken in all the liquid and become tender. Five minutes from the end of cooking add all the fish and give it a good stir once again. Leave to cook for a further 5 minutes.

5. Serve with extra steamed vegetables.

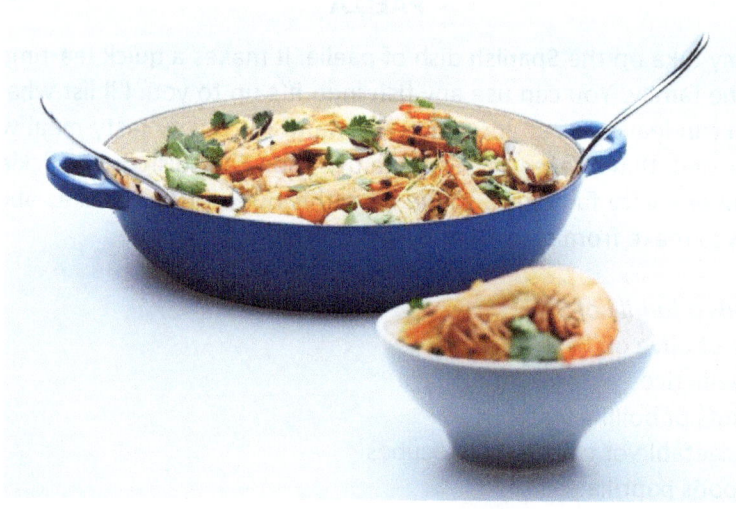

HONEY MUSTARD AND CHICKEN PASTA

I like making different pasta dishes, especially at the moment as I'm training for my runs and I need carbohydrates for extra energy, endurance and stamina. I love pasta recipes that are really easy to make and that are healthy too; I don't want to make anything that's stodgy and slows me down. All the family love a good pasta dish.

Serves 4
10oz/300g farfalle or any other pasta shape
3 tablespoons reduced-fat mayonnaise
1 heaped teaspoon wholegrain mustard
1 teaspoon clear honey
10oz/300g cooked chicken, torn into rough pieces
4 spring onions, thinly sliced
4 tomatoes, quartered
Salt/pepper

1. Boil the pasta following the packet instructions, and then cool under cold running water.

2. Mix the mayonnaise, mustard and honey in a large bowl and loosen with a splash of water to make the dressing the consistency of double cream.

3. Add the cooked pasta, chicken, spring onions and tomatoes. Season then gently mix together.

4. Serve on a bed of green salad.

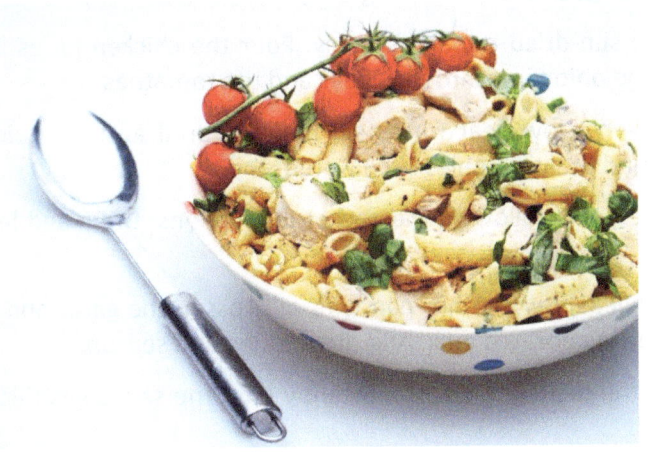

PENNE PASTA WITH CHICKEN AND SUN DRIED TOMATOES

The sun-dried tomatoes in this recipe really gives it a smoky, intensely flavourful taste. You'll know exactly what I mean when you make it.

Serves 4

¼ jar of sun-dried tomatoes, rinsed and patted dry on kitchen paper
6oz/175g skinless chicken breasts, cubed
¼ cup of white wine
1 tablespoon dried Italian seasoning
1 onion, peeled and sliced
2oz/50g mushrooms, sliced
½ cup frozen peas
7oz/200g dried penne pasta
5 garlic cloves, peeled and crushed
1 tablespoon plain flour
360ml evaporated milk
1/8 teaspoon ground nutmeg
½ teaspoon chilli powder
1 tablespoon fresh basil, chopped
5 black olives, thinly sliced
Salt/pepper

1. Preheat the oven to 180C/350F/Gas mark 4.

2. Combine the chicken and wine in a shallow baking dish. Sprinkle the Italian seasoning on top. Bake for 20 minutes until the meat is no longer pink in the middle and the juices run clear. Remove from the oven and shred the warm chicken, reserving the juices for later.

3. Slice the sun-dried tomatoes thinly. Pour the chicken juices into a large pan. Add the onion, mushrooms, peas and the tomatoes.

4. Sauté over a low heat for a few minutes until all the liquid has been absorbed and the vegetables have wilted.

5. Cook the pasta following the packet instructions. Drain and leave to one side.

6. Meanwhile, spray another pan with oil. Toss in the garlic and flour, then whisk in the evaporated milk. Add the nutmeg and season.

7. Reduce the heat and whisk constantly until the sauce has thickened. Stir in the basil.

8. Transfer the cooked pasta to a serving bowl. Add the chicken, vegetables and sauce. Toss together and garnish with the sliced olives and serve.

CORN CHOWDER

Serves 4
Light oil cooking spray
1 onion, peeled and chopped
2 large tins sweetcorn
700ml chicken stock (fresh or made up with boiling water and 2 chicken stock cubes)
1 red pepper, deseeded and finely chopped
½ teaspoon fresh rosemary, chopped
½ teaspoon dried thyme
Cayenne pepper to taste
1 teaspoon fresh basil, chopped
Salt/pepper

1. Spray a large pan with oil and heat. Sauté the onions for about 4 minutes or until translucent.

2. Add the corn and stock and bring to the boil. Turn down the heat and simmer.

3. Add the pepper and all the herbs, season and simmer for 5 minutes.

4. Transfer the contents of the pan to a blender and puree until smooth. Return to the pan and turn the heat off. If it looks a bit thick, either add a little more stock or hot water. Serve with shredded steamed vegetables – try to choose vegetables in an array of different colours to make sure you're getting all the different nutrients and vitamins needed for a healthy diet.

CHICKEN ROGAN JOSH

Here's one of my recipes for a healthy curry without calories! Well, there's no such thing as that, but this recipe has less oil in it, and is therefore more healthy for you. I hope you like it. I've been making this curry all my married life, it's my own healthy curry recipe, and we think it resembles a chicken rogan josh. Curry connoisseurs out there might beg to differ!

Serves 2
2 chicken breast fillets, diced
A dash of olive oil
1 onion, peeled and chopped
3 cloves garlic, peeled and finely chopped
6 button mushrooms, sliced
1 tin chopped tomatoes
1 squeeze of tomato ketchup
1 dessertspoon medium curry powder
1 heaped teaspoon turmeric
1 teaspoon cumin
1 dessertspoon chicken gravy granules
Splash of water
Salt/pepper
Optional ingredients: half a butternut squash, peeled and cubed, or 1 red pepper, sliced.
2 portions of pilau rice cooked according to the instructions on the packet. Whilst cooking the rice I always add 1 heaped dessertspoon medium curry powder, 1 teaspoon turmeric and a handful of sultanas, then I microwave cook the rice – I find it much easier.

1. Fry off and seal the chicken, onions, mushrooms and garlic in a dash of olive oil for a few minutes or until the chicken turns white on the outside and the onions are translucent and soft.

2. Add the tinned tomatoes, spices, gravy granules, tomato sauce, red pepper, and the butternut squash if using it. Give it a good stir and turn the heat down to a low simmer. Season well.

3. Simmer for at least 10 minutes or until the chicken is cooked (and the butternut squash soft). It might need a splash of extra boiling water at this stage if you think the consistency is too thick.

4. With a teaspoon check the heat of the curry by tasting it. Everyone's palate is different; if you like it hotter then add more curry powder and carry on simmering for a few more minutes.

5. Serve straight from the pan on your spiced pilau rice. Enjoy!

CHICKEN OR BEEF STIR FRY

I love this dish because it's dead simple. You can even add a few more healthy bits and pieces if you like. It takes about 15–20 minutes to make from start to finish, and saves you slaving for an hour over the oven. It's also full of healthy tummy filling goodness too. You will need a very big pan or wok though. I don't actually own a wok and my frying pan isn't large enough to stir everything evenly, so I use my big soup pan instead, it works just as good.

Serves 4/5
Splash of olive oil
2 pieces of frying steak or 2/3 skinless chicken breasts, cut up into strips
2 inch piece fresh ginger, peeled and grated
2 teaspoons brown sugar
3 tablespoons dark soy sauce
3 tablespoons white wine vinegar
1½ tablespoons tomato ketchup
2 teaspoons cornflour
600g bag mixed stir fry vegetables from any supermarket
1 bag of fresh noodles
1 bag beansprouts
1 red onion, peeled and sliced
3 cloves garlic, peeled and finely chopped
6 mushrooms, sliced
1 tin water chestnuts
Salt/pepper

1. Start by heating a large frying pan or wok on a high heat with a splash of olive oil, add the beef or chicken.

2. Fry for approximately 5 minutes or until your beef/chicken is nearly cooked.

3. Add the onion, mushrooms and garlic and fry for a further couple of minutes or until the onion has turned translucent. Add the mixed stir fry vegetables and water chestnuts, then cook on for a further 4–5 minutes. Add the fresh noodles at this stage, always making sure you're stirring continuously.

4. In a small bowl mix together the cornflour, white wine vinegar, tomato ketchup, brown sugar and soy sauce until it makes a smooth paste.

5. Peel and finely grate the ginger into the paste and stir, leave to one side. You're probably better making the paste at the beginning of the cooking so it leaves your hands free to stir the pan continuously.

6. Add the beansprouts to the pan and give it a very good stir.

7. Once everything is in the pan add the paste mixture and stir continuously until it thickens slightly, this should take about 2 minutes. Season well.

8. Serve straight from the pan and eat while it's still hot. This dish is not that good heated up again, it really needs to be eaten fresh. In saying that, my hubby eats this dish reheated when he gets home late from work and he absolutely loves it.

SALMON AND PRAWN SALAD AND SPICY SLAW

A great meal, it has to be said. It's certainly one of my favourites. It's a salad so any salad vegetables go. I accompany it with my bursting with flavour spicy slaw. I love any type of salmon; the one I use for this meal has already been cooked and flavoured so it saves precious time and effort when you need a quick meal, and this is "my" type of ready meal.

Serves 2
2 sweet chilli salmon fillets – you will find them in any large supermarket along with the fresh prawns, mackerel, crab stick etc. They are readily available in two-portion packages
1 bag fresh/frozen medium prawns
1 bag of mixed salad leaves or any lettuce, plus cherry tomatoes, cucumber, red onion, sweetcorn, red pepper, celery etc – anything that you like on a salad

For the Spicy Slaw

½ red cabbage, peeled and thinly sliced
1 white onion, peeled and thinly sliced
3 carrots, peeled and grated
3 tablespoons of low fat mayonnaise
1½ teaspoons chilli powder
2 tablespoons whole grain mustard
2 tablespoon sweet chilli sauce – all good supermarkets sell this on the sauces aisle
Salt/pepper

1. Start by making up a nice-sized salad on a dinner plate. Fill it with all your favourite salad vegetables. Top with a piece of salmon with the prawns placed around the each salmon fillet.

2. Now to make the spicy slaw. Thinly slice the red cabbage and onion, grate the carrots, or prepare in a food processor to save time, then put into a large mixing bowl.

3. In a separate bowl add the mayonnaise, wholegrain mustard, sweet chilli sauce and chilli powder. Mix well.

4. Add the mayonnaise sauce to all the vegetables and stir well. This can be kept in an airtight container in the fridge for up to a week.

5. Add a serving spoon of the spicy slaw to the your salad and season if necessary.

THREE BEAN CHILLI CON CARNE

This dish is great to make in advance to eat the next day or you can freeze portions so that you always have a healthy meal to pop in the microwave and have ready in minutes.

Serves 4
500g lean minced beef
1 onion, peeled and chopped
6 mushrooms, sliced
3 cloves garlic, peeled and chopped
1 large tin reduced sugar baked beans
1 large tin red kidney beans, rinsed
1 large tin cannellini beans, rinsed
A squirt of tomato ketchup
3 tablespoons Worcestershire sauce
1 heaped tablespoon beef gravy granules
2 teaspoons medium chilli powder
A splash of boiled water
Salt/pepper
6 large steamed carrots to accompany this dish or other steamed vegetables. If you wanted something a little more substantial you could try serving it with a small portion of brown rice or a jacket potato.

1. Heat a large pan but DO NOT add any oil. Now dry fry the mince, onions, garlic and mushrooms until slightly browned, stirring all the time.

2. Turn the heat down and add the baked beans, kidney beans, cannellini beans, tomato ketchup, Worcestershire sauce, chilli powder and gravy granules. Season and stir well. At this stage, if you think it's too thick add a splash of water to the pan and stir.

3. Place a lid on the pan and cook on a slow heat for 10–15 minutes. Before serving, taste to check if the chilli is hot enough in flavour; add more chilli powder if required, and stir.

4. Serve on a bed of steamed carrots or any other steamed vegetables you like, or accompanied by a small portion of boiled brown rice.

CHAPTER 13

Healthy Snacks

Obviously it's up to you how much you eat of these and how often you have them. My rule of thumb is always be sensible – a palm full of each listed item is enough as this is a snack and not a meal. There are some very good calorie counted and low fat snacks available in supermarkets, but be careful because they can leave you wanting more and sometimes don't really leave you satisfied. Also they're not always quite as good for you as the manufacturers make out, so check the fat and calorie content. I always think you can't go wrong with making your own snacks so you know exactly what the contents are.

- Mixed nuts and raisins.
- Olives.
- Cooked chicken chunks or pieces (preferably steamed).
- Chopped carrots (as many as you like of these).
- Pot of low fat yogurt.
- A piece of fruit, i.e. apple, orange, banana, grapes, plums, strawberries, blueberries.
- Dessertspoonful of low fat cottage cheese on a dry Ryvita.
- One slice of my home-made banana cake.
- One of my home-made carrot muffins without the frosting on top.
- Three rice cakes. I love rice cakes. They're good on a couple of levels. First, they don't have many calories, so you can have more than one at once. Second, they take ages to eat because of their size and texture. In the supermarket you will find lots of different flavours too. My favourite are the savoury ones, and the cheese ones are tasty. My kids love them too, so they're great for all the family to munch on for a healthy snack choice.

- Healthy fresh fruit yogurt. That's easy-peasy! My family and I are big fans of these yogurts as a pudding. You can add any fresh or dried fruit depending on what you like. The kids can really get involved too and it teaches them about choosing a healthy option dessert. Into each bowl, we add 2 dessertspoons of low fat Greek yogurt or a normal low fat natural yogurt, and add a few pieces of chopped fresh fruit in any combination. This can be apple, banana, peach, pear, pineapple, melon, kiwi, plum, grapes, strawberries, blueberries, raspberries, orange etc. To this, we add some dried fruit, e.g. raisins, sultanas, goji berries, cranberries, banana, apricots, dates. Then we add a handful of mixed nuts and 1 teaspoon of runny honey. Finally, we like to top our yogurts off with a dessertspoon of grape nuts for extra texture and taste. You will find grape nuts in the cereal aisle of any good supermarket. To me, they taste just like crushed up biscuits, but they are not, they're a crunchy wheat and malted barley cereal.

- One flapjack square.

- Below are two of my healthy flapjack recipes.

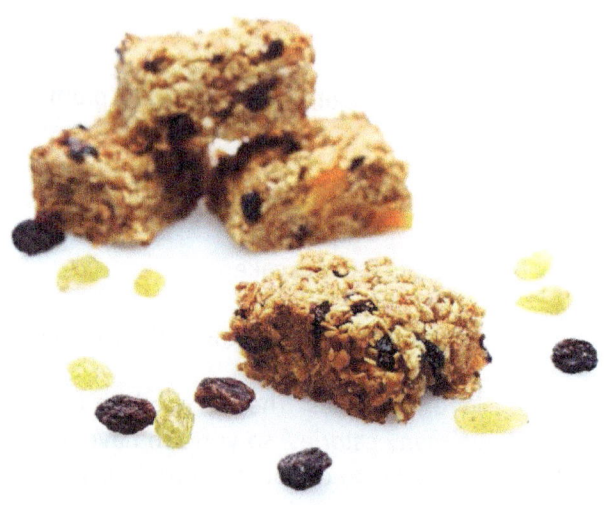

HEALTHY FRUITY FLAPPY JACKS

8oz/225g honey
8oz/225g porridge oats
8oz/225g granola
8oz/225g brown sugar
4oz/110g butter or margarine
2oz/50g extra dried fruit (any of the following: sultanas, raisins, currants, apricots, cranberries, dates)

1. Place the butter, honey, brown sugar and the extra dried fruit into a pan and melt down. Simmer for about 5 minutes on a low heat.

2. Place the porridge oats and granola into a bowl and pour the liquid ingredients over the top.

3. Give it all a good stir until everything is well coated.

4. Grease a 20cm x 30cm baking tin and pour in all the ingredients. Firmly press down and push into all corners of your tin.

5. Place in a pre-heated oven at 170C or equivalent for 20 minutes or until golden brown all over.

6. Leave to cool for approximately 5 minutes, then cut into squares with a very sharp knife. Remove from the tin with a fish slice or similar implement. Enjoy, and don't forget – the smaller you cut your squares, the less the calories are in your flapjack. You should be able to cut 15 squares out of the whole tray bake.

HEALTHY HONEYED FLAPPY JACKS

3oz/75g brown sugar
3 tablespoons honey
12oz/300g porridge oats
3oz/75g dried apricots
1 small ripe banana

1. Place the brown sugar and honey in a pan and slowly heat through then simmer for 2 minutes.

2. Place the porridge oats and apricots in a mixing bowl and stir through.

3. In another bowl mash up the ripe banana with a folk until it looks like baby food and is totally combined.

4. Add the warm honey and sugar to the oats, mix well then add the banana and mix again until it's all combined.

5. Grease a 20cm x 30cm baking tin. Spoon in the mixture, press it down, push it into all four corners and flatten off.

6. Place in a pre-heated oven at 170C or equivalent for 20 minutes or until golden brown all over.

7. Remove from the oven and leave to cool for about 5 minutes before cutting into 15 pieces with a sharp knife. Remove from the tin. If left too long in the tin you may find they are a little difficult to remove.

CHAPTER 14

Soups

SPICY BUTTERNUT SQUASH SOUP

This is one of my all time favourite soup recipes. I could just live off this soup, it's so full of goodness, is very tasty with not many calories and packed with nutrients. This quantity makes a large pan full. I make this amount so it lasts the week, kept in the fridge in an airtight container to maintain the freshness, for quick ready-made lunches. Don't tell anyone, but it was Michael Winner's favourite soup too. I made it for him on many occasions.

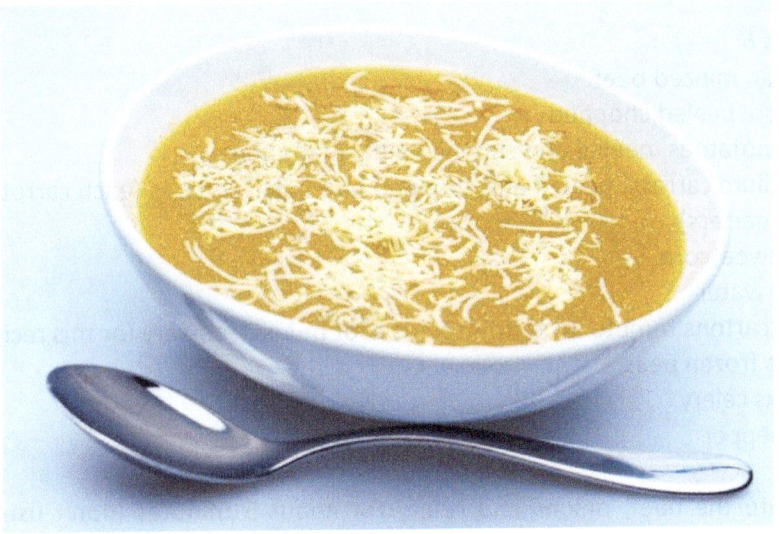

Serves 8–10
4 large or 5 small butternut squash, peeled and cubed
8 teaspoons of cumin
3–4 pints water
4 chicken stock cubes
6 garlic cloves, peeled and chopped
4 onions, peeled and sliced
Salt/pepper

1. Peel and roughly chop the onions. Peel the butternut squash and remove all the seeds and cube all the flesh. Peel and chop the garlic.

2. Put everything into a large pan, add the water, chicken stock cubes and cumin. Bring to the boil and simmer for about 10–15 minutes or until all the vegetables are tender. Season well.

3. Turn off the heat and either liquidise or blitz with a hand-held blender.

BEEF AND VEGETABLE SOUP

This is a very meaty soup with a thick consistency; a little stew really, and a good winter's evening family tea that also very filling. This is great warmed up the next day, or portioned off and frozen for a later meal.

Serves 6
1lb lean minced beef
1 onion, peeled chopped
6 red potatoes, peeled and chopped into small cubes
4 medium carrots, peeled and chopped into small squares (each carrot ring into quarters)
1 tin sweetcorn
½ cup water
1½–2 cartons tomato juice (this seems a lot but is necessary for this recipe)
2 cups frozen peas
3 sticks celery
Salt/pepper

1. Sauté the beef, onions and celery for about 5 minutes (don't use any extra oil), and season well.

2. Add the carrots and potatoes. Turn the heat down and add the rest of the ingredients.

3. Simmer for 20 minutes then serve.

CELERY SOUP

Another great soup that freezes really well too.

Serves 2–4
A splash olive oil
350g celery, washed and chopped
2 cloves garlic, peeled and chopped
1 red onion, peeled and chopped
14 fl oz water
3 chicken stock cubes
Salt/pepper

1. Heat the oil and fry off the onion and garlic until translucent; this takes approximately 4–5 minutes.

2. Turn the heat down and add the water, stock cubes and celery.

3. Simmer for 10–12 minutes then turn the heat off. Blend with a hand blender or liquidiser until smooth.

PUMPKIN SOUP

This is a great soup and not just at Halloween. It's a great way to use up all the flesh from inside your carved pumpkins – this was the reason I came up with this recipe; I was fed up with all the waste. I have three kids so that's an awful lot of pumpkin insides not to make use of. Have no fear, this recipe is "Perfection Personified".

Serve 4
1 large pumpkin
2 onions, peeled and roughly chopped
1 teaspoon cinnamon
½ teaspoon nutmeg
1.7 litres/3 pints water
3 chicken/vegetable stock cubes
2–3 cloves of garlic, peeled and chopped
Salt/pepper

1. Start by cutting the top off the pumpkin with a sharp knife.

2. With your hands or a spoon, scrape out all the seeds and discard.

3. With the spoon start scraping all the flesh from around the sides, making sure not to go through the outside skin – well, that's only important if you're thinking about carving the pumpkin for Halloween!

4. Spoon all the flesh straight into a large pan. Add the rest of the ingredients and bring to the boil, then turn down and simmer for 10 minutes. Season well.

5. Turn the heat off and liquidise with either a liquidiser or handheld blender until smooth.

CARROT AND CORIANDER SOUP

I love carrots – they're not just for rabbits. Carrots don't just have to be boiled up and served as a vegetable, they can be used in ways that make them centre stage. Carrots make amazing soups and cakes!

Serves 4
450g carrots, peeled, washed and chopped
1 onion, peeled and chopped
1 heaped teaspoon coriander
1 large white potato, peeled and cubed
1.2 litres water
3 chicken/vegetable stock cubes
Handful of fresh coriander
Salt/pepper

1. Except for the fresh coriander, add all the ingredients to a large pan and bring to the boil. Season and simmer for 20 minutes.

2. Liquidise and add the fresh coriander, either do this in a food processor or with a hand held blender.

3. Serve straight from the pan whilst still hot.

TOMATO AND BASIL SOUP

This is a great recipe because I use tinned tomatoes instead of fresh, so they're already prepared. All that roasting off and deseeding and skinning, you can do it but it takes time, and in this day and age time comes at a high price – not everyone has a lot of it. I also like the fact tinned tomatoes are cheap to buy, cheaper even than fresh, and because the taste is still there, you'd struggle to tell I hadn't used fresh tomatoes in this soup. So this all adds up to a cheap and cheerful choice for me. This soup also keeps really well in the refrigerator for up to a week, and freezes well too. Easiest soup ever!

Serves 4
3 large tins of chopped tomatoes
1 onion, peeled and sliced
3 clove garlic, peeled and chopped
½ pint water
1 chicken/vegetable stock cube
Large handful of basil leaves, roughly chopped
Salt/pepper

1. Add all the ingredients to a large pan. Bring to the boil and simmer for 15 minutes, season well.

2. Whiz everything up in a blender until it's smooth.

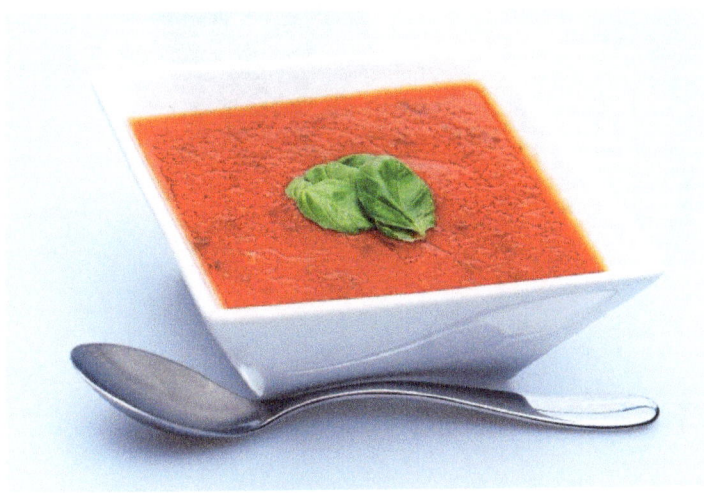

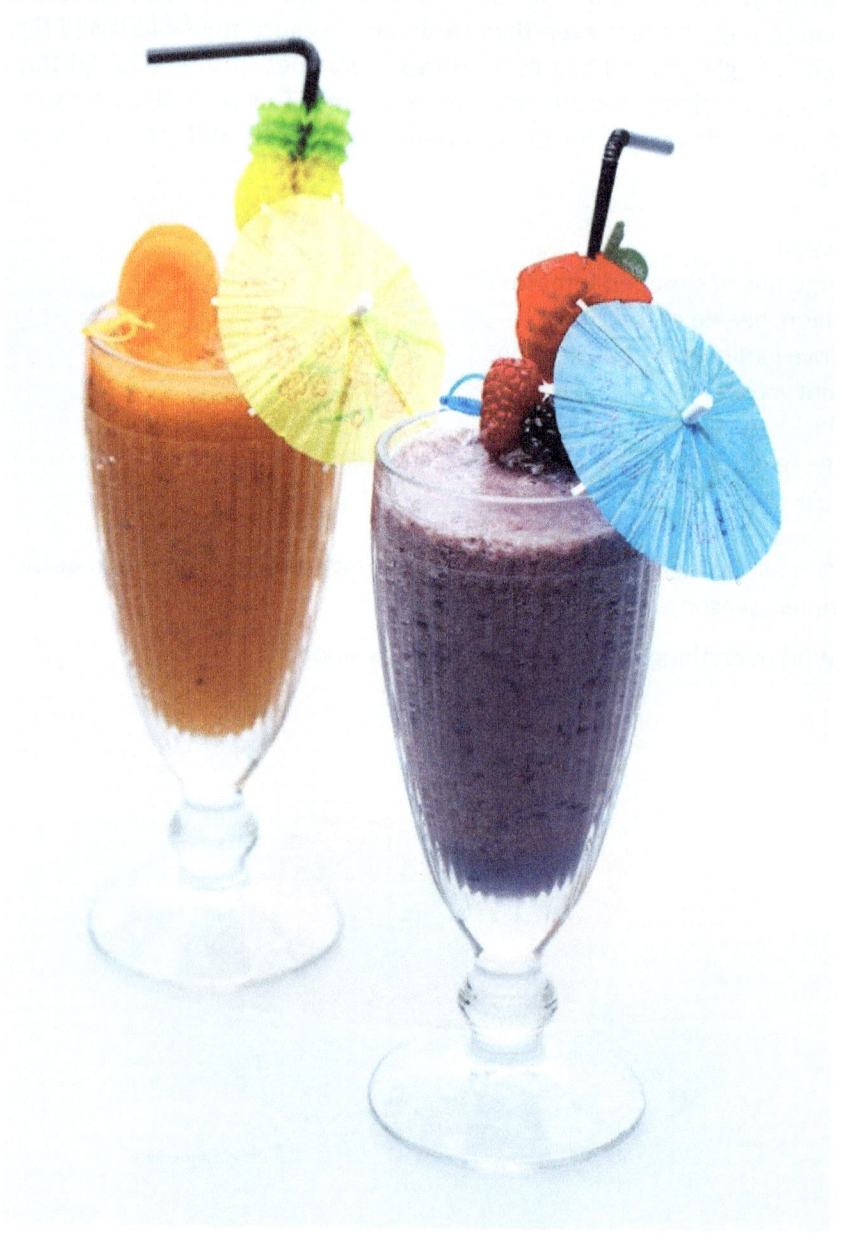

CHAPTER 15

Super Smoothies

I love a good smoothie. These home-made ones are what I had for my lunch every day for the first 6 months on my Plan. You can have them for a meal replacement or just a snack. They're crammed packed with healthy foods to give you that boost of energy and keep you going through the day. They're all very easy and quick to make – all you need is a smoothie machine or a liquidiser. My smoothie recipes are all one serving.

THE ENERGY BOOSTER

This smoothie is packed with vitamins A, C, K, and B12 to perk you up instantly and to boost your immune system.

4 peeled carrots
1 apple, unpeeled
1 kiwi fruit, peeled
Handful of parsley
Extra water if you think it's too thick

Place all the above ingredients into a smoothie liquidiser and blitz; you may find you have to chop your carrots up a little before liquidising them. Smoothie machines vary so much depending on how much you pay. Usually the cheap ones aren't that good at liquidising everything up. When you're using carrots or nuts they seem to get stuck with the machine constantly stop–starting. Before buying one, I would recommend looking at the various models around for the machine that's best for you. Just remember, the dearest ones aren't always the best ones.

THE SEXY SMOOTHIE

This one will get the blood flowing to all the right places. It will even boost testosterone to bring out the tiger in you.

400g strawberries
225g cherries
1 tablespoon grape nuts (you can find them in the cereal department of any good supermarket)

Blend all the above. You can also add some crushed ice or some cold water to this one if you find it a little thick.

THE HEALTH WARRIOR

A miracle cure it isn't, but this smoothie has all the ingredients that are known to help prevent the likes of liver, lung and colon cancer. This is a good one to take on your travels for the day. Just keep it somewhere cool, and shake it back to life when you want it.

100g blueberries
Half a water melon
I small pot of natural low fat yogurt
2 tablespoons muesli
1 orange

Peel and dice the water melon, then add everything and blend together.

THE BRAIN BOOSTER

Essential fats, vitamin B6, glucose, tyrosine. Blend them all together and you've got the solution for a sharper mind and more mental alertness.

100g blueberries
50g strawberries
1 banana
2 teaspoons peanut butter
2 tablespoons flaxseeds (you can get them from any good health food shop or large supermarket)
1 small pot of low fat yogurt (any variety or natural)

Blend everything together with a couple of ice cubes and enjoy.

THE MOOD LIFTER

Rich in potassium, folic acid and vitamin B, all of which will raise your spirits and help put a smile on your face. This one is really good as a lunch or tea substitute as it tastes like a cold soup.

2 peeled carrots, diced up small
1 beetroot
1 red pepper, deseeded
Handful of fresh parsley
Some extra ice cold water as the consistency of this one can be quite thick.

Blitz together and enjoy!

THE EXERCISE BOOSTER

Packed with antioxidants to fight the radical damage of training, it will replace lost energy. This is also a very good one to take on your travels in a cooler box/pack.

300ml skimmed milk
50g blueberries
50g blackberries
1 banana

Blitz all together and enjoy either before exercise or after, for that extra boost.

THE FAT BUSTER SMOOTHIE

Low in calories, high in nutrients and filling enough to stop you reaching for the biscuits. This is also a very good meal replacement smoothie, and kept in a cool place it travels very well also.

6 tomatoes
2 celery sticks
140g natural low fat yogurt
100g low fat cottage cheese
Splash of Worcestershire sauce
Handful of fresh parsley

Blitz altogether until smooth. It can be quite a thick consistency, so add some extra cold tap water if needed.

THE HANGOVER SMOOTHIE

This will soothe a dicky tummy, replace lost minerals and is simple enough for even the fuzziest of heads to make the morning after.

3 apples, unpeeled
2 carrots, peeled
A small chunk of peeled and grated ginger
Some extra cold water

Blitz all the above together and serve.

THE BODY BOOSTER

Helps to restore a tired body and helps strengthen bones. Altogether more effective than a magic wand!

1 avocado
1 papaya
200ml low fat natural Greek yogurt
1 red chilli, deseeded
1 banana
1 slice of pineapple

Peel and dice all the fruit and the chilli. Blitz altogether in your liquidiser until smooth. Add a splash of cold water if you think it's a little too thick.

Tips when making smoothies
The ones with banana, apple or pear in have to be drunk immediately after being made, as the fruit in them separates and goes brown. Don't make these ones in advance as they do not travel well. Also make up ones yourself; don't stick religiously to any of my recipes. Add honey to sweeten if necessary and you could add oats and pine nuts to bulk them out if you're using them as a meal replacement.

Yogurt, milk and water are good not just for the taste but also for making smoothies smooth.

Fruit juice is also good for making them smooth. I use a lot of apple juice in mine (sugar free, of course). I don't tend to make a lot with oranges or satsumas because I don't particularly like the taste and I think it overpowers everything else you put in. Always remember, if you think they look a little too thick, just add some cold tap water to thin down.

Make your own recipes up, they really are so easy. All you need is some kind of liquidiser, food processor, hand held blender or a proper smoothie maker. They range from cheap and cheerful to very professional and expensive. You can use milk, water, ice, yogurt or, for a special treat, ice cream to make your smoothies extra smooth. Then all you have to do is add any of the things listed below.

Bananas (they are quite fattening so I tend not to use a lot of them), apples, pears, kiwi, grapes (red or green), melon (any variety), peaches, lemon, lime, apricots, plums, raspberries, blueberries, strawberries, blackberries.

Remember, when you make a smoothie with bananas, pears or apples, you do need to drink them straight away.

To sweeten a smoothie I always use honey but you could try a flavoured yogurt instead of using a natural one.

For savoury smoothies try mixing together a couple of the following vegetables. All should be used raw; don't pre-cook them as they are much better for you as none of the vitamins have been cooked out.

Tomatoes, carrots, beetroot, spring onions, celery, cucumber, spinach, fresh herbs, courgettes, sweetcorn, peas, green beans, chilli, ginger.

Now it's your turn to have a play around and experiment with flavours that you like.

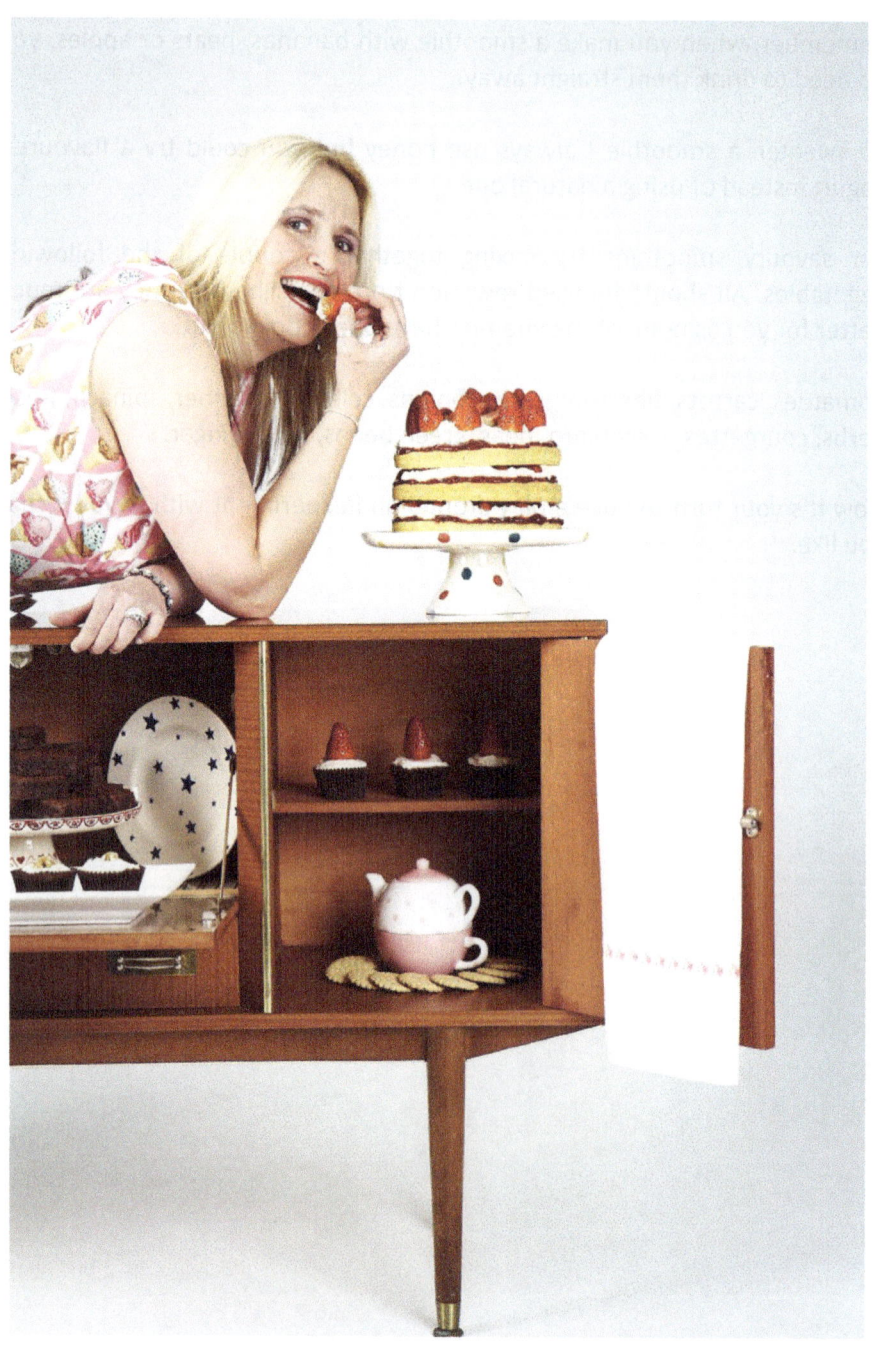

CHAPTER 16

Cakes and Puddings

In this chapter I'll start off with my four favourite "healthier" cake recipes. These are the same four cake recipes that I have written into Chapter 7: The Plan. These are the cakes I've used throughout my two-week meal/food plan. In fact, three of them I've always made, even before my journey began and I was morbidly obese. I still make these and eat them with great pleasure, the only difference being nowadays I cut a smaller piece or only eat one scone or muffin at a time, unlike when I used to demolish whole family-size cakes to myself.

Cakes and pudding always contain a certain amount of sugar and fats, that's what makes them so scrumptious, and I love muffins! Muffins are great when you need to control the portion size you're eating. They're already the right size to eat as they come in individual portions thus less chance of cutting such a massive slice or eating the whole cake. Always remember that cakes and puddings do contain calories and you should always be aware that eating too much of a good thing isn't necessarily good for you. On the other hand, life without cake would be no life at all! Personally, I need a sweet kick regularly; depriving myself would only mean total disaster for me, for that's when sticking to a healthy plan can get boring and when there is more chance of not succeeding in maintaining a healthy lifestyle.

BANANA CAKE

My favourite cake of all time! I can't remember where or why I started eating it, but it's been on our family's favourite treat list for literally years and years. I make this cake as presents for friends a lot too. I demonstrate this recipe quite often at food festivals. I also love it because it's such a simple recipe and it's all measured in cups – no messing around with kitchen scales. Everyone seems to like my banana cake, even people who don't like bananas will regularly come up after sampling it to tell me they're a convert. It's a very moist cake, so you don't even need butter on it, and it's simply perfect with a brew. It lasts up to two weeks in an airtight container or you could double all the quantities given and make two banana loaf cakes and freeze one.

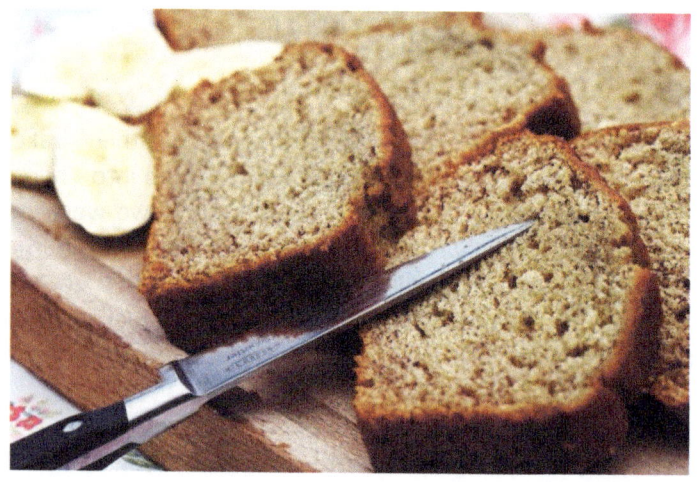

3 over ripe bananas (the blacker the better)
1½ cups plain flour
1 teaspoon of vanilla extracts
1 teaspoon bicarbonate of soda
½ teaspoon of baking powder
1 dessertspoon of butter or margarine
1 cup of sugar
1 egg

1. Whiz all the above ingredients except the flour in a food processor until it's all smooth. If you don't have a food processor you can do this in a bowl with a hand held mixer, or with a fork and lots of elbow grease. Start by forking the bananas if you're doing it this way until well mashed, then slowly add the rest of the ingredients.

2. Add 1½ cups of plain flour to the rest of the ingredients. If you're doing it by hand or in food processor always add the flour after everything else has been well mixed in. Whiz everything until combined and then pour into a greased and lined loaf tin.

3. Bake in a pre-heated oven for 45 minutes on 170C or equivalent. Remove when baked and leave to cool before slicing and serving with a nice hot brew. Delicious!

BRAN CAKE

I have my good friend "Parky" – one of my running friends and gym buddies – to thank for this recipe. She's been making it for years and passed the recipe on to me. I have altered the quantity of sugar used, though, as for me, it was too sweet. See what you think. Again, this recipe is great because everything's measured in cups and there's no butter/margarine in it what so ever – BONUS!

1½ cups All-Bran (don't use any cheap cereal brand, it has to be the proper stuff)
1½ cups whole milk (again, I wouldn't recommend skimmed or semi with this recipe)
1 cup sugar
2 cups sultanas
1½ cups self raising flour

1. Soak the All-Bran with the milk, sugar and sultanas for at least an hour or until all the ingredients have soaked up the milk.

2. Add the flour and give it a good old stir.

3. Place in a greased and lined loaf tin and bake in a pre-heated oven 160C or equivalent for 50–60 minutes.

4. Once cooked, removed from the oven and leave to completely cool before slicing.

This cake keeps for up to two weeks in an airtight container, and freezes well too.

CARROT MUFFINS

I absolutely love these babies; tasty, naturally sweet and very moist. My hubby, Chris, actually prefers them unfrosted and they have less calories in them that way, and are equally good without it. I would suggest making in batches and freezing them separately unfrosted, ready for when you need a sweet, healthy treat. These are great to make with children to get them involved in cooking and baking, a great way to show them how to make healthy food from scratch and how to include a vegetables in cake baking. Kids love making and eating these. These are also one of my favourite cakes to demonstrate at food festivals and they always go down a storm with the general public.

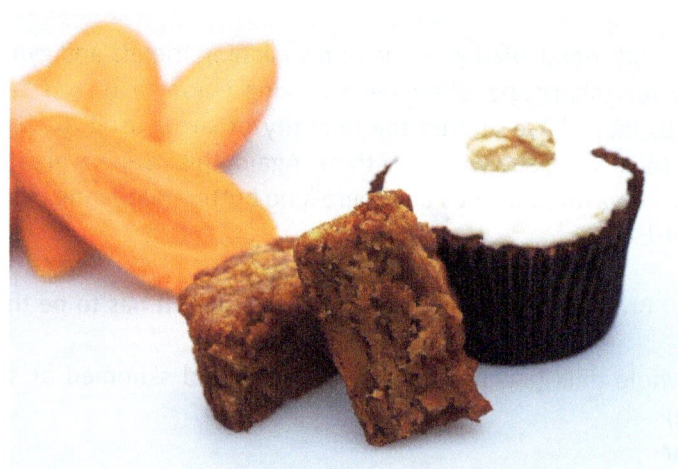

Makes approximately 15 muffins
10 oz/280g plain flour
1 teaspoon baking powder
1 teaspoon bicarbonate of soda
2 teaspoons ground cinnamon
1 egg
3 fl oz milk
2 tablespoons runny honey
4oz/110g granulated sugar
3 large carrots, peeled and grated on the largest size grate
1 teaspoon vanilla extract
3 fl oz vegetable oil
Optional: a handful of chopped walnuts or sultanas

1. Pre-heat the oven to 180C or equivalent and place muffin cases in the muffin tin.

2. Into a large mixing bowl, sift together all the dry ingredients.

3. In a measuring jug mix together all the wet ingredients.

4. Add the peeled and grated carrots to the dry ingredients. If you are using optional walnuts or sultanas, add at this stage. Mix well so all the grated carrot is coated in the flour etc.

5. Now add all the wet ingredients and give it a really good mix until everything is well combined and it resembles a thick batter mixture.

6. With two dessertspoons, evenly divide the mixture between all of the muffin cases, roughly two spoonfuls in each one.

7. Place in a pre-heated oven for 20 minutes, or until golden brown and springy on top to touch.

8. Remove from the baking tin and place on a wire rack to cool.

Cream cheese frosting for the carrot cake – optional

2 oz/50g low fat cream cheese at room temperature
6oz/175g icing sugar
½ teaspoon vanilla extracts

1. Place all the above (no need to sift the icing sugar) into a mixing bowl and mix together with a fork. At this stage you'll think "no way will all this amount of icing sugar combine to make a soft frosting." But it will, have patience.

2. Once it's all come together and there are no lumps in it, frost your cakes evenly. This amount will frost one whole batch.

No licking the bowl though – just think of all those extra calories!

MY BASIC SCONE RECIPE

These are very basic and easy to make. I used to love making these in my children's cookery class at school. Warm out of the oven, and filled with jam and whipped cream, all the teachers loved sampling the fruits of the morning's cookery lesson. You just can't beat our fine traditional delicacy that is the English scone. I always put sultanas in mine; you don't need to and some people even say it's a sacrilege if you're filling them with jam (and if you're not being good, freshly whipped double cream too). If you're making batches, I would strongly recommend freezing them separately ready for using them in your meal plan, as they don't keep very well and go hard and crusty in no time at all. Top thumb note for this recipe – Best is fresh!

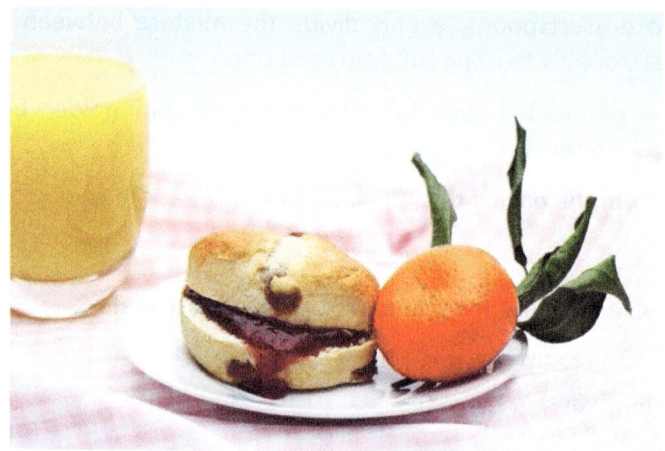

1. Pre-heat the oven to 220C or equivalent. Lightly grease two baking trays.

2. In a mixing bowl add the flour and sugar and mix. Then add the margarine and mix together with your fingertips to form breadcrumbs (rubbing in).

3. Then add the milk and bring it all together like dough.

4. Turn out onto a floured surface and split into 10 even sized pieces.

5. Roll each piece of dough into a ball shape (try not to overwork it as it will become tough).

6. Place five on each baking tray and press the tops down slightly with your fingers to make them look a little flatter, brush with a little milk.

7. Bake in the oven for about 8–10 minutes or until golden brown on top.

8. When cooked, remove from the baking tray and leave to cool on a wire rack.

9. When completely cool, bag up most of them separately and freeze until needed.

The rest of my cakes and dessert selection is what it is! I've chosen a selection of some of my favourite recipes. Of course they're not calorie free, but you have to be sensible about it. All the way through my weight loss journey I made these for my family for their puddings and treats. I didn't eat them; this is the part of "YOUR" journey where willpower will kick in. Just because you're cutting down and swopping some foods for more healthier options, that doesn't mean the rest of the family has to be so strict on themselves about what they eat, especially if they haven't got the pounds to lose. Everything in moderation! I know from first-hand experience by the way I was brought up, that making things into BAD/NAUGHTY foods and never being allowed them, makes you want them even more. That's when you can find yourself overdosing on them because you never know when you might get to try them again. Well, that was certainly the way with me. My family is being brought up to try all different foods. Some naughty but nice, and some healthy for you. We live off a very varied diet where no food is a sin. It's all about how much of it you eat. The size of your portion not the type of food, is what it's all about.

CHOCOLATE BROWNIE LOAF CAKE

I'm obviously not going to give you my famous Chocolate Brownie recipe; if I did that I would only have to kill you! This recipe is exceedingly good though. I've been making it such a long time, in fact years before I discovered my award winning Chocolate Brownie recipe. This amount makes two loaf tin cakes.

10oz/300g plain flour
1 teaspoon bicarbonate of soda
3oz/75g cocoa powder
500g caster sugar
10oz/300g margarine or butter
3 eggs
2 teaspoons vanilla extract
120ml sour cream
200ml boiling water
10oz/300g good quality dark chocolate roughly chopped

For the syrup glaze

2 teaspoons cocoa powder
250ml water
8oz/225g caster sugar
2oz/50g quality dark chocolate

1. Cream together the sugar and margarine/butter. You can do this either in a big bowl with a wooden spoon, or in a food processor. Add the cocoa powder, bicarbonate of soda, eggs, vanilla extract, flour and sour cream. Bring everything together then add the boiling water slowly. If you're using a food processor, turn down the machine and add the water slowly through the funnel at the top.

2. With a spatula place all the mixture into a mixing bowl and add the chocolate chunks. Combine all the chocolate mixture well into a thick lumpy batter.

3. Grease and line two loaf tins and split the ingredients between them.

4. Place in the oven on 170C or equivalent for 1 hour, test with a skewer to check if the inside is cooked enough, if not leave for a further 5–10 minutes.

5. Ten minutes before the end of the baking time, place all the glaze ingredients into a heavy bottomed saucepan and bring to the boil. Turn down and simmer for 10 minutes, this reduces the glaze down to make it thick and sticky.

6. When the chocolate brownie cakes are done remove from the oven and prick all over with a toothpick to make holes everywhere. Pour over the glaze, the holes will help the glaze to soak into the cakes and make them moist.

7. Leave to cool in their tins.

These cakes will last up to two weeks wrapped up in an airtight container, or you could freeze one of them for another day.

STICKY TOFFEE CAKE

Our favourite pudding in a cake, this is a real winner! A really great moist cake, and it also keeps well. Plus, I love the way you top the cake with the sticky sauce instead of making a big jug and pouring it over (overdosing on the calories). So in effect, this is portion controlled. Again, it's another one of my recipes which you can eat without the sticky topping – it's certainly just as good and saves so many calories too.

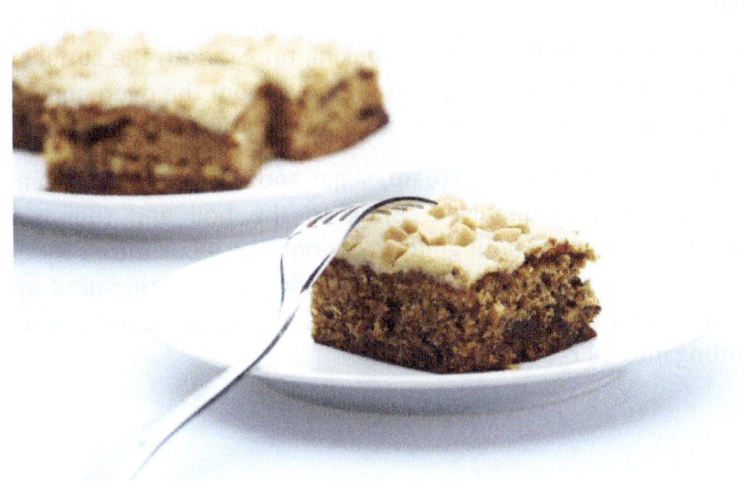

8oz/225g dried dates
300ml of water
1 tsp bicarbonate of soda
6oz/175g soft light brown sugar
4oz/110g butter, room temperature
1 tsp vanilla
2 eggs, beaten
6oz/175g self raising flour

The toffee icing

3oz/75g soft light brown sugar
1oz/25g butter
2oz/50g icing sugar, sifted
6 tablespoons fresh double cream

1. Preheat the oven to 180C/350F. Butter and base line a shallow 11 x 7 inch baking tin. Set aside.

2. Cut each date in two. Place in a saucepan along with the water. Bring up to the boil, and then boil uncovered for about 10 minutes, until all the water is absorbed and the dates have softened. Remove from the heat. Stir in the bicarbonate of soda and set aside to cool.

3. Cream together the butter and brown sugar. Stir in the vanilla. Gradually beat in the eggs and then fold in the slightly cooled date mixture. Finally, stir in the flour.

4. Spoon the batter into the prepared baking tin. Smooth the surface. Bake for 25 minutes, until risen and just set. Remove from the oven and leave in the tin for 15 minutes before turning out onto a wire rack to cool.

5. For the icing, gently heat the cream, sugar and butter together in a small pan until the sugar is dissolved. Bring to the boil and then simmer, uncovered for 4 minutes, until golden. Do not stir. Pour into a Pyrex dish and when it's nearly cooled add the sifted icing sugar stirring until smooth. Using the back of a wet spoon, spread the icing over the cake. Leave to set before cutting into 18 rectangles.

To find out more about Justine Forrest and her online bakery visit: www.browniesbyjustineforrest.com.

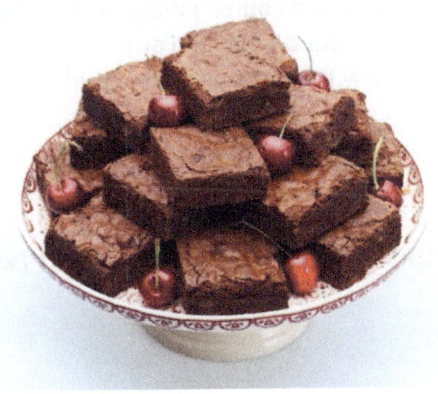

Praise for Justine's Brownies

"Historic beyond belief, a taste experience – perfection!"
Michael Winner

"Bloody lovely" Sir Roger Moore

"Better than sex!" Ted Robbins

"Cooked from the heart…" Giorgio Locatelli"

"A real find" Andrew Neil

Website: www.justineforrest.co.uk
Facebook www.facebook.com/justine.b.forrest
Twitter https://twitter.com/JustineForrest

Justine Forrest teaches cookery courses at **The Wellbeing Farm** - a lovely cookery school in a relaxing environment, where you can learn how to lose weight and make healthy recipes.

To book a course please visit:
The Wellbeing Farm
www.thewellbeingfarm.co.uk

Look out for *Justine's Journey Part Two*

If you have enjoyed this book, please take a moment to write a review, no matter how brief, on Amazon and/or GoodReads or send ThornBerry Publishing a comment via our website www.thornberrypublishing.com. Authors value and appreciate readers' feedback.

Thank You

Lightning Source UK Ltd.
Milton Keynes UK
UKOW06f0142231113

221635UK00012B/42/P